Precision Livestock Farming

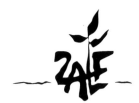

Centre for Agricultural Landscape and Land Use Research (ZALF)
Eberswalder Strasse 84
D-15374 Muencheberg
Germany

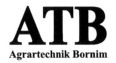

Institute of Agricultural Engineering Bornim (ATB)
Max-Eyth-Allee 100
D-14469 Potsdam
Germany

Precision Livestock Farming

Edited by
S. Cox

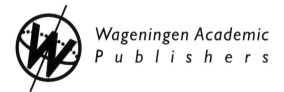

Wageningen Academic
P u b l i s h e r s

CIP-data Koninklijke Bibliotheek
Den Haag

ISBN 9076998221

paperback

Subject headings:
precision livestock farming
information systems
livestock management

First published, 2003

Photo cover:
Andreas Jarfe

Wageningen Academic Publishers
The Netherlands, 2003

Printed in The Netherlands

Scientific panel

Herman Auernhammer	Germany
John Bailey	Great Britain
Franz Josef Bokisch	Germany
Reiner Brunch	Germany
Sidney Cox	Great Britain
Richard Dewhurst	Great Britain
David Filmer	Great Britain
Andy Frost	Great Britain
Rony Geers	Belgium
David Givens	Great Britain
Henk Hogeveen	Netherlands
Pieter Hogewerf	Netherlands
Anders Jonsson	Sweden
Thomas Jungbluth	Germany
Peter Kettlewell	Great Britain
Joachim Krieter	Germany
Jos Metz	Netherlands
Toby Mottram	Great Britain
Dieter W. Ordolff	Germany
David Parsons	Great Britain
Wim Rossing	Netherlands
Lars Schrader	Germany
Bart Sonck	Belgium
Jack Whittier	USA
Gavin Wood	Great Britain

Reviewers

Thomas T. Amon	Joachim Krieter
Daniel Berckmans	Tadeusz T. Kuczynski
Franz-Josef Bockisch	F. Madec
Reiner Brunsch	Jos J. Metz
Wolfgang Büscher	Soren Marcus Pedersen
Andreas Fischer	Bart Sonck
Gates	Herman Van den Weghe
Jacobson	C.E. Van´t Klooster
Anders Jonsson	J.A.M. Voermans
Thomas Jungbluth	Eberhard von Borell
Otto O. Kaufmann	Georg Wendl

International program committee of the 1st ECPLF

Organizers
Prof. J. Zaske, (ATB, Germany)
Dr. A. Werner, (ZALF, Germany)

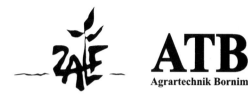

Editors of the ECPLF Proceedings
Sidney Cox (UK)

Country representatives for ECPLF
A. R. Frost, (UK)
R. Kaufmann, (Switzerland)
K. Sallvik, (Sweden)
Prof. Dr. Ir. Daniel Berckmans, (Belgium)
Dr. Ir. Cees van't Klooster, (Netherlands)
Dr. Soeren Pedersen, (Denmark)

Program Committee

Prof. Juergen Zaske,	Institute of Agricultural Engineering Bornim (ATB), Potsdam-Bornim
Dr. Armin Werner,	Centre for Agricultural Landscape and Land Use Research, (ZALF), Müncheberg
Prof. Herman Van den Weghe,	Georg-August-University Göttingen, Vechta
Prof. Hermann Auernhammer,	Weihenstephan Center of Life and Food Sciences, Freising-Weihenstephan
Prof. Eberhard von Borell,	Martin Luther University Halle, Halle/Saale
Dr. Jens-Peter Ratschow,	Association of Engineers, Münster
Dr. Detlef Ehlert	Institute of Agricultural Engineering Bornim (ATB), Potsdam-Bornim
Dr. Reiner Bruinsch	Institute of Agricultural Engineering Bornim (ATB), Potsdam-Bornim
Dr. Andreas Fischer	Centre for Agricultural Landscape and Land Use Research, (ZALF), Müncheberg

Conference Office of the 4ECPA and 1ECPLF

Andreas Jarfe	Centre for Agricultural Landscape and Land Use Research, (ZALF), Müncheberg

Contents

Editorial

As far as I am aware, this is the first international conference on Precision Agriculture principles that has featured livestock farming. The European ECPA series - like those elsewhere around the world - stemmed from the application of the NAVSTAR Global Positioning System, which enabled farmers to acquire yield maps automatically at harvest time, and hence to apply site-specific treatments to land and crops.

It can be (and has been) argued that small farmers have employed PA for millennia, through their intimate knowledge of local variations in their fields. Nevertheless, they did not possess the range of measurement tools that we now have, nor the capacity to model their processes that is provided by today's digital computers.

The same situation has existed in livestock farming but this sector of agriculture has not (yet) been transformed by a single technical development, comparable to GPS. Instead, over the past quarter of a century PLF has become established through animal specific developments of several kinds, notably transponders for animal identification (now coded to ISO standards); automatic animal weighing (now an application of image analysis); methods of controlled feed rationing and, lately, robotic milking. There is now ample evidence that livestock farmers will adopt new technology if it meets their needs to provide high quality products in the most economic ways. Public concerns for animal welfare and for the traceability of an animal's life history have further broadened the scope for PLF, since they involve both animal- specificity and site- specificity.

With these aspects of traceability and control of process quality in production, both precision technologies share the same goals, as well as similar scientific methods and scientific principles in the process context. But without doubt these are not the only areas of common methodology, or of similar or identical technical solutions. Many aspects in scientific research of PA and PLF are related almost identically to (i) systems research and modelling of complex systems, (ii) explaining (production) process performance by complex sets of interacting driving forces, (iii) variability in space and time as a basic feature of data and information, (iv) designing concise data models and minimum datasets in information processing, (v) enhancing the basic research data of process understanding with evidence based information or from on-farm research, (vi) decision making with complex but limited information under uncertainties, (vii) information management on different complexity levels in the farm: from the separately distinguishable object in the production management (sub-part in the field, single animal in the flock) over object-aggregates (fields, crop rotations, flocks, herds) to whole farms.

Many aspects of economic or ecological-impact analysis from agricultural activities on fields or with the livestock can only be determined when defining a joint system-border. Thus limiting the scientific research to one of these strands is mostly not feasible. At least it would result in too limited answers to actual scientific and societal questions.

The Organising Committee of 1ECPLF therefore made a creative and far-sighted decision to associate 4ECPA with 1ECPLF. Furthermore, a first attempt was made to specify what we mean by PLF, through the selection of the ten Conference themes.

The number of papers submitted to the meeting is undoubtedly somewhat disappointing, but this is compensated by wide coverage of the Conference themes. Much of the work presented is at an early stage, too. Nevertheless the potential of PLF is established. It is to be hoped that Berlin 2003 will provide the starting point for regular coincident (if not combined) meetings at which subjects of common crop and animal interest can be promoted.

Sidney Cox
Editor

A proposal for an "Agrar BUS" as a Farm Area Network

R. Artmann

Institute of Production Engineering and Building Research, Bundesallee 50, D-38116 Braunschweig, Germany

Abstract

A standard solution is needed for the non-uniform manufacturer networking of agricultural computer systems. Due to the anticipated exponential growth of the Industrial Ethernet, agriculture should also use this technology. A close linking of "agricultural standards" to an established industrial standard is recommended. Based on Ethernet IP/TPC and UDP, a concept for an "Agrar BUS" is presented. Here a middleware is responsible for the network services and communication to the applications, and a web based document exchange serves as the basis for a uniform user interface. Both the equipment and the data objects are mapped with XML. A rapid standardisation under the auspices of the ISO is recommended.

Keywords: Agrar BUS, Ethernet, Networking, Bus in Agriculture, Computer Systems

Introduction

For an optimal orientation and implementation of production, a recognition of the links between the areas of production, marketing, administration and information access and processing, as well as environmental concerns, is becoming increasingly important. The information flow is not limited to the farm or the production, but is increasingly networked with external information sources and recipients. Automatic milking systems, for example, can only be implemented in a sensible way if the fastest possible rectification of disturbances can be achieved through direct connection with the service provider. On-line connections are in part adequate for diagnosis and perhaps also for the elimination of problems. This type of assistance will also become standard for other types of computer controlled systems.

A standard for the networking of the farm internal economy must be able to carry out all required data transactions between all electronic components which make data available (data sources) and/or require data (data recipients). Not only the networking in animal husbandry should be covered, but also storage, ventilation, relationship, sales, source of information, and information distribution (external farm communication) as well as to external electronic systems (ISO 11783, Weather and Weighing Station, etc.) The necessity for this networking stems from economic, ecological and animal welfare aspects.

In this paper, a concept for a standard will be presented, optimally defined at the international level (ISO). It is based on author's work (Artmann 1986 and 2000) development trends in industry (Kriesel et al. 2000, Furrer 1998), and is the discussion basis for the working group "BUS farm internal economy," and now as a basis for the "New Work Item" (ISO7TC23/SC19 N210 Stationary equipment for agricultural and forestry - communications data network for livestock farming) to be voted upon.

Technological trends and the status of networks in agriculture and industry

Four trends of information technology are significant in the future development of computer controlled systems in agriculture:
- in terms of hardware, increasingly inexpensive "embedded PCs" or pre-fabricated modules are being implemented

- in terms of software, graphic programming, projection and simulation by manufacturers is becoming increasingly important
- the complexity of systems requires on-line diagnosis and updates, through to external maintenance
- a complete networking of devices should permit the general availability of all desired data in the entire enterprise and permit connections to intra- and internet.

Computer controlled systems used in animal production limp, particularly for devices which are since longer time on the market, behind these trends. The hardware is mostly based on self-production, programming takes place with machine languages, external maintenance use an analogue modem, and networking includes in the best of cases the components of one manufacturer. For the redesign of these equipments the newest technology shall be used.

The increasing pressure to rationalise production requires a quick, efficient and comprehensive availability of all relevant data from an enterprise, and in addition information about competitors, market, etc. This pressure has led to the situation that "Industrial Ethernet" is today seen as "the solution" for a comprehensive networking in an enterprise. But is unfortunately still the case that the large producers of field bus systems remain inflexible and the innovations come from smaller, more agile companies.

The concept

The lack of existing BUS systems and the preference as well as the enormous availability of Ethernet in the office world, with the related price drops for modules and components which led to the wish to use Ethernet in production.

An IDA (Interface for Distributed Automation) group and an ODVA (Open Device Vendor Association) exist for the industrial sector. These two groups are allied under the umbrella group IAONA (Industrial Automation Open Networking Alliance). The IAONA has the goal of establishing a worldwide standard for the use of Ethernet in every industrial environment. There should be an interface free communication about all areas of the enterprise (www.iaona-eu.com). Developments in industry have led to the facts that the non-deterministic Ethernet has now up to a microsecond real time ability and the rough environment conditions are handled through different protection classes (IAONA 2002).

There is no sense in agriculture reinventing the wheel. It is much more important to adapt industrial developments in an efficient and inexpensive way, and to develop new products only when there are no alternatives. Under consideration of general technological trends, the industrial development and performance as well as the status of the networking in agriculture was recommended by the author in 2000 (Artmann 2000) Ethernet and TCP/IP as significant components of a worldwide standard for the future networking in agriculture. It is based on the industry suppliers offering exclusive inexpensive modules with Ethernet interface with scalable performance ability (type and amount of inputs and outputs, storage and processor capacities etc.) for the field level, which cannot be made individually because the costs of developing hardware, and at this time, also software, would be prohibitively expensive.

In order to use this module for agricultural purposes without problems, it is necessary to keep the agricultural standard as close as possible to the industrial standard. With the decision to use Ethernet and the protocols IP, TCP/UDP only the OSI levels 2 to 4 are specified (Volz 2000). A need for norming exists for the Physical Layer and for everything which is settled between the Transport and Applications Layer. Suggestions are listed below:

Physical layer

The Physical Layer deals with the topology of the network, the laying of cables, socket and active components. Here, a second draft from the IAONA is available (IAONA 2002) which makes the topology shown in Figure 1 possible. Two environmental protection classes, "light duty" for the installation in protected cases (IP 20) or rather "heavy duty" for the direct integration in an industrial environment (IP 67) are established as are the specifications for copper and fibre optic cables for 100 MHz as well as sockets with RJ-45 or rather M12-faces.

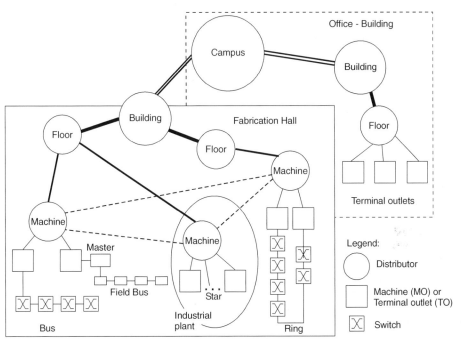

Figure 1. Topology of the backbone arrangement for an agriculture net (according to IAONA 2002).

The IAONA specifications could be taken over by agriculture. In some cases, stricter regulations would be necessary by the usage temperature as well as resistance to moisture, aggressive gases and damage from rodents.

For the connection to mobile units (PDA's, feed mixing wagons, etc.) but also as an interface to the external economy (ISO 11783, Tractors and Implements) the specifications of a radio network liked to the Ethernet are recommended. Wireless LAN according to IEEE 802.11b in 2,4 GHz ISM Band were already used together with the industrial Ethernet (Siemens 2001, Gergeleit and Schumann 2002, Meyfarth and Lohmann 2002). For use areas in which only minimal transfer distances are required or in some cases a localisation of, for example, the user, the chances for "Bluetooth" (Anonymous 2002) must be evaluated and defined perhaps in combination with the network. This technology is particularly interesting due to the low costs and the automatic findings.

The middleware

With a computer system distributed across the entire enterprise, with components from different manufacturers, the task of the Middleware is to make possible the complicated programming of the network and to offer high performance tools for the exchange of data, for network configuration, management and service. This means that both a thorough definition of the data structures as well as equipment specifications are needed. The protocols Ethernet, IP, TCP, and UDP are not appropriate to be used for the development of general applications. The do build, however, the basis for higher protocol levels. In commercial applications, protocols like FTP, Telnet, NFS, HTTP, CORBA, DCOM, and others, which make the link between the transport Layer and the real application, Figure 2. It is proposed that the agricultural standard be leaned closely on the specifications of the IDA group (IDA 2002). The reasons for this are: it is an open source, the solutions are innovative and it is already in use.The following central elements shall be realised:

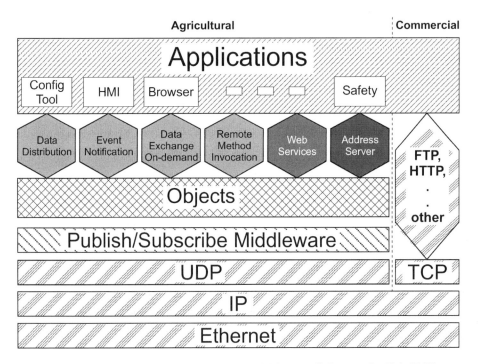

Figure 2. Communication services for an agricultural Ethernet (following the IDA 2002).

1. General definition of the devices (equipments) and the data as **objects** *and their description with Extensible Markup Language (XML)*

Each device which can be attached to the Ethernet BUS contains a generally valid exact description of it's origin, for management (configuration and control) as well as the integrated functions and applications, similar to a printer driver. A similar approach is used for profibus applications. The description of the device is content in the Device Type Manager (DTM). The DTM is created and delivered with the device by the manufacturer. With Engineering Tools (Field

Device Tool (FDT) the DTMs are readed and automatically integrated into the network. Open source products are available, for example: PACTware (www.pactware.com).

Data and data pacts shall be defined as objects via XML schemas. This is one of the most difficult and comprehensive tasks. Here though the data dictionary can be built according to ISO 11788. Helps for the conversion of data into XML and back are under development (Paulsen 2002). The application of the full potential of would make the program too wieldy for small applications. For this reason, the use of a compiler and parser is recommended with limited ability, for example, no dynamic schemas, no validation, replacement of DOM and SAX Application Interfaces (API) through data transfer in simple C structures (Gordon 2002). Agriculture has the opportunity here to describe principally the objects with XML schemas, to convert them before use in the network according to ISO 11788, and to communicate internally only in this format.

2. *Uniform object oriented name space*

It is proposed to develop the name space hierarchically according to the network topology. A clear name for a device is given through the linking of the hierarchy levels to the device. With the structure shown in Figure 1, the following *name* is used to "Machine Outlet x" **//CD.BD$_a$.FD$_b$.MD$_c$.MO$_x$**, where C, B, F, M, MO represent Campus, Building, Floor, Machine and Machine Outlet, a, b, and c are the correspondent unit.. Through the linking with the subsequent structure, the individual device will be reached.

Data objects are addressed with subsequent "/" without further details (all objects) or with object names (for example, status//CD.BD$_a$.FD$_b$.MD$_c$.MO$_x$/**status**) or rather object and element names (//CD.BD$_a$.FD$_b$.MD$_c$.MO$_x$ /**status.temperature**).

Methods (services) following the device names are linked with a ".", for example //CD.BD$_a$.FD$_b$.MD$_c$.MO$_x$.**set**.

3. *Data exchange with a Real Time Publish/Subscribe Protocol and general Services*

The IDA group specified for this task NDDS from RTI (Pardo-Castellote et al., 2001, IDA 2002). This protocol, in its current form, sets requirements which are too high for the device resources. These should, however be made scalable, so that they can be used in an embedded system. The advantage of this protocol is the not targeted communication. The publishers place their information in the network and subscribers pick them up as needed. With four API services (data distribution, event notification, data exchange on demand and remot method indication), compare Figure 2, it is possible to create a comfortable data exchange. The Middleware must be capable of dealing with other problems as well, such as redundant publishers. For a detailed description of see the User Handbook (RTI 2000) and the IDA specifications (IDA 2002).

4. *Generally valid Human Machine Interface (HMI) via WEB Browser*

Particularly in agriculture, where mostly one person must deal with very different computer systems, the simple, easy-to-learn and uniform service a common HMI for all systems is of special value. This is all the more important, because some systems are only used occasionally or with greater time spans. The use of XML to define objects is in conformance with the further development of Hypertext Markup Language (HTML) which will also use XML. The devices can exchange data via a XML capable server applications (i.e., Simple Object Access Protocol (SOAP)). This must be possible to realize an automatic documentation of processes and material flows through the whole production (Birkhofer and Russ 2001, Kunitz 2002). The integration of the HMI based on WEB browser in DTM and engineering tools, like FDT, is necessary. Further significant requirement for the Middleware are:

5. *Services for configuration, management and network.*
6. *Compatibility with the communication via TCP and commercially used protocols*
7. *Processes for the clock synchronisation of participants for real time tasks.*

For point seventh, there are also IDA specification available for these tasks. So that true real time would be possible with Ethernet. IEEE 15888 specifies a process for the synchronisation of clocks of the BUS participants (Jennings 2002). Also the integration of a time server into the switches (Holmeide and Jakob 2002) is a possible solution

Conclusions

Just one, comprehensive all-inclusive networking system encompassing the existing interdependencies and an optimal controlling of production with consideration of the needs of animals and environment is needed for agriculture for many reasons. In addition, the system must be capable of providing a reliable and credible documentation of all production methods. This is a factor of ever-increasing importance in the acceptance of agricultural products by consumers.
A standardised solution is needed for the networking of agricultural computer systems from different manufacturers. Due to the expected exponential growth of Industrial Ethernet in industry and for use in the appropriate protocols in all offices, intra and internet application, agriculture should hop onto this train.
There are already IDA specifications for an open source standard for Industrial Ethernet. They could serve as a basis for the standards to be developed for agriculture. A framework for these standards is presented. It is necessary that the drafting of an ISO Norm take place quickly. Here it is particularly important that the decisions for the standards be based on future and not on present possibilities. The information technology is still very innovative. Even if some of its features appear illusory in three or four years, and that is how long it takes to publish a standard, the Utopia could hopefully be exactly right.

References

Anonymous 2002. Drahtlose Zukunft. Bluetooth in der Industrie. [Wireless future. Bluetooth in the industry.] Messtec & Automation (10) 52-53.
Artmann, R. 1986. A Proposal for Physical Link and Data Link Control for Interfacing Computer Systems on Farms. In: Agri-Mation 2. Chicago. 224-234.
Artmann, R. 2000. Informationstechnologie in der Innenwirtschaft. [Information technology in the interior economy.] KTBL-Schrift 390 15-20.
Birkhofer, R: and Russ, M. 2001. Internet-Technologie auf Automatisierungskurs. [Internet technology on automation course.] IEE (S1) 32-34.
Furrer, F.J. 1998. Ethernet-TCP/IP für die Industrieautomation. [Ethernet TCP/IP for industrial automation.] Grundlagen und Praxis., Heidelberg.
Gergeleit, M and Schumann, R. 2002. Funk-WLAN und Echtzeit. [Radio WLAN to and real time.] IEE (S1), 100-103.
Gordon, Ch. 2002. XML for Device Networking and Communications. http://ethernet.industrial-networking.com/articles/i09xml.asp and .../i10.asp.
Holmeide, Ø. and Jakob, M. 2002. Ethernet-Switch mit Zeit-Server. [Ethernet switch with time server.] IEE (4) 66-69.
IAONA 2002. Industrial Ethernet Planning and Installation Guide. Draft 2.0, Magdeburg, 59 pp.
IDA 2002: Architecture Description and Specification. Rev. 1.1, Blomberg,
ISO 11783. Tractors and machinery for agriculture and forestry Parts 1-11.

ISO 11788. Electronic data interchange between information systems in agriculture Agricultural data element dictionary. Parts 1-3.

Jennings, S. 2002. IEEE 1588 - die Synchroniosation über Ethernet. [IEEE 1588 - the synchroniosation over Ethernet .] IEE (7) 52-55.

Kriesel, W. Heimbold, T. and Telschow, D. 2000. Bustechnologien für die Automation. [Bus technologies for automation.] 2nd Ed. Heidelberg.

Kunitz, H. 2002. Bindeglied für die vertikale Integration. [Link for the vertical integration.] IEE (1) 32-33.

Pardo-Castellote, G., Thiebaut, S. S., Hamilton, M. and Choi, H. 2001. Real-Time Publish-Subscribe Protocol for Distributed Real-Time Applications. http://www.rti.com.

Paulsen, Ch. 2002. Bundesinitiative EDI-AGRAR. [Federal initiative EDI-AGRAR.] www.lkv-wl.de/frame/adis-aded/praesentation.

Meyfarth, R. and Lohmann, W. 2002. Kleine Bedienung für Unterwegs. IEE (1) 34-35.

RTI, 2000. NDDS User´s Manual, Version 2.3. Real-Time Innovations, Inc. CA.

Siemens 2001. Industrielle Kommunikation in neuer Dimension - mit Industrial Wireless LAN. [Industrielle communication in new dimension - with industrial wireless LAN.] Firmenunterlage Nr.E2001-A50-P820.

Volz, M. 2000. Wegweiser durch den Protokollstack. [Guide through the protocol stack.] CSMA/CD-Buszugriff. Internetprotokoll, Transportprotokolle TCP und UDP. In: Praxis Profiline. Industrial Ethernet. 16-19.

Acknowledgement

The represented contents were partly discussed in the German working group "bus inside economics" and are based partially on their results.

Results of continuous measurements of ear temperature in boars

J. Bekkering[2], H. Brandt[1] and T. Hoy[1]
[1]*Justus-Liebig-University Giessen, Department of Animal Breeding and Genetics, Bismarckstreet 16, D-35390 Giessen, Germany*
[2]*Cooperation for Promotion of Pig Housing, Zum Pöpping 29, D-59387 Ascheberg, Germany*

Abstract

Fifty-one singly penned boars in an artificial insemination station were included in the analysis. Each had a special ear tag with a temperature sensor. Ear-skin temperatures were measured every 3 min. A typical diurnal daily rhythm of ear temperature with the lowest value in the morning and a peak in the afternoon was observed in the boars and monitored up to 136 days with 96 measurements each day. The results of 210 measurements from 42 boars, including 16 boars with increased rectal temperature (≥ 39.3 °C = fever), showed that the coefficient of correlation between skin and rectal temperatures is small (r = 0.31).

Keywords: boar, rectal temperature, skin temperature, fever.

Introduction

In the future, there will be more regulations in the EU member states concerning monitoring and documentation of the health status in animal production. The outbreaks of foot and mouth disease (mainly in UK) and of European swine fever during recent years together with the growing size of livestock production unit have shown the importance of fast and sound information on the actual health situation in farms. So, animals showing first symptoms of a disease can be treated as soon as possible. Artificial insemination (AI) stations with boars are the centre of interest because of the increasing extent of AI in swine in Germany and in other countries. In consequence, the hygienic risk of transmission of infectious diseases including epidemics via semen transport is rising. It is nearly impossible to measure the rectal temperature of boars in AI stations daily because hundreds of boars are kept in several stations. Over more than 25 years different non-invasive infrared temperature measurements have been tested (Roehlinger et al. 1979, 1980). But, these authors as well as Zinn et al. (1985) have not used continuous measurements of skin temperature. In our own investigations, it was necessary to adapt and develop a specific system of automatic measurements of ear temperature in boars as an early warning. The aim of our investigation was
- to test the computer supported system QSS 2000 (QSS = quality safety system - W. Scheffelke, Diatech GmbH, D-26970 Walchum, www.qss2000.de) for continuous measuring of ear temperature in boars kept in AI stations and
- to analyze the possibilities of these continuous skin temperature measurements to detect clinical signs (esp. rising rectal temperature) of boars.

Materials and methods

Fifty-one boars of different breeds (mainly Pietrain) singly penned in one house of an AI station were included in the analysis. The pens measured 6 up to 7.5 m^2. Each had a concrete floor with straw as bedding material. The boars were fed twice a day with concentrated feed. Semen was collected once or twice a week. Beside the semen collection all treatments due to a disease were registered in the AI station.

The boars carried a special ear tag with a sensor covered in plastic material. The sensor with a temperature resolution of 0.02 °C, calibrated by Diatech GmbH and an absolute accuracy of

0.5 °C measures the skin temperature at the ear every 3 minutes and creates a mean temperature on the basis of five 3-minute values. These means were automatically transferred via an aerial to a computer with the QSS 2000. The software generates a continuous curve of dynamics of the ear temperature for each boar. Additional information about the individual animals (e.g. rectal temperature, treatment, semen collection) can be added into the programme. On the PC screen all boars measured are shaped as little pigs with individual numbers. Upper and lower bounds of warning temperature can be set. If the temperature curve of one animal crosses the upper or lower bound a warning signal is shown on the screen and the colour of this individual on the PC screen is changed from green to red or blue for high and low temperatures. The data are stored in an Access data base and can be exported to other programmes like Excel or SPSS for statistical analysis. Two sensors were installed in the boar house (each at a height of approximately 2.3 m) to continuously record the room temperature.

The skin temperature of the left ear was continuously measured from December 2001. Due to problems with some sensors not all boars were monitored during the whole year. The rectal temperature of 42 boars was measured with a digital thermometer 5 times after vaccination against influenza on November 6, 2002. The first measurement was between 1.5 and 3 hours after vaccination (between 8.50 and 10.16 a.m.), the next 6 hours later. The third measurement took place next morning (between 5 and 6 a.m.) followed by another measurement in the afternoon (between 3 and 4.30 p.m.). The last measurement of rectal temperature was two days after vaccination. This period was chosen because a rise in rectal temperature was expected after the vaccination. The rectal temperatures were merged with the nearest single and one-hour averages of the skin temperature and summarized in an Excel file. Using SPSS for Windows 8.0 the descriptive statistics for all parameters and the coefficients of Pearson's correlation were calculated.

Results

From 57 to 136 days with 96 measurements each day in 5 boars analysed we observed a typical daily rhythm of the ear temperature with a drop in temperature in the early morning (between 3 and 5 a.m.) and a peak in the afternoon (between 3 and 5 p.m.) (see an example in Figure 1). At the moment those 5 boars are a random sample vicarious for the whole group. During the night the standard deviation of the ear temperature was much higher (up to ± 5.8 °C) than during the afternoon (between ± 2.0 and 2.8 °C). Shortly after semen collection a small rise in ear temperature with large individual differences between boars was measured, but no differences in the mean ear temperature between the days before, at and after semen collection were found.

The mean rectal temperature of 42 boars after vaccination against influenza (a total of 210 measurements) was 38.1 °C with a standard deviation of ± 0.9 °C. The minimum was 35.4 °C and the maximum 40.5 °C. Approximately 6 hours after vaccination 18 boars had fever (rectal temperature ≥ 39.3 °C). In 3 boars the fever was permanent up to the next morning. Two boars were treated with 20 ml Metamizol each because of remaining high rectal temperature after vaccination. The ear temperature did not show a clear rise in all boars. The single values (15 min-means) and the one-hour-means of skin temperature at the left ear were nearly the same. The average of the skin temperature ranged from 20.9 °C (15 min-value) to 21.0 °C (hour-means) (Table 1) showing a large variation. The standard deviation (for all 210 values) was 4.7 °C, 4.5 °C resp. with a minimum of 12.1 °C, 13.1 °C and a maximum of 31.9 °C, 34.1 °C resp. The room temperature during these approximately 48 hours was on average of 14.9 ± 0.7 °C with a minimum of 13.5 °C and a maximum of 16.2 °C.

The coefficients of correlation between the rectal temperature and skin temperature at the ear (based on 15 min-single-value and 1 hour-mean next to the time of measuring rectal temperature) were low and ranged between 0.31 and 0.32 ($p < 0.01$) (Table 2). That means that approximately 10 % of the variation of the ear temperature can be explained by the change in rectal temperature.

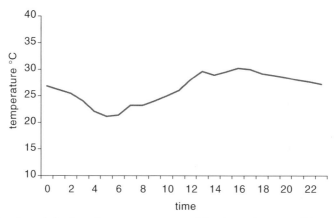

Figure 1. The diurnal rhythm of ear temperature of five boars between 56 and 136 days.

Table 1. Descriptive statistics of rectal temperature, skin temperature at the ear of 42 boars at 5 terms after vaccination against influenza and of room temperature in the boar house (n = 210 measurements).

	mean (°C)	standard deviation (°C)	minimum (°C)	maximum (°C)
rectal temperature	38.1	0.9	35.4	40.5
skin temperature 1	20.9	4.7	12.1	31.9
skin temperature 2	21.0	4.5	13.1	34.1
room temperature	14.9	0.7	13.5	16.2

1 - 15 min-value next to the time of measuring the rectal temperature
2 - 1 hour-mean next to the time of measuring the rectal temperature

Table 2. Coefficients of Pearson correlation between rectal temperature, skin temperature at the ear of 42 boars at 5 terms after vaccination against influenza and of room temperature in the boar house (n = 210 measurements).

	skin temperature 1	skin temperature 2	room temperature
rectal temperature	0.31	0.32	0.49
skin temperature 1		0.91	0.36
skin temperature 2			0.42

1, 2 see Table 1. All coefficients $p < 0.01$

The relationship between room temperature and rectal temperature ($r = 0.49$, $p < 0.01$) seems to be closer than those between ear temperature and rectal temperature. This led to an analysis of the dynamics of the ear temperature of one boar during 147 days with 3519 values in dependence on room temperature. If the room temperature was higher by 5 °C the mean ear temperature was also higher by nearly the same value (Table 3).

Table 3. Mean ear temperature for a boar in dependence on room temperature.

room temperature °C (from ... to)	mean room temperature (°C)	n	ear temperature (°C)			
			$\overline{x}$	± SD	Min	Max
15 ... ≤ 20	17.6	2234	24.9	± 4.8	14.2	36.4
> 20 ... ≤ 25	21.5	1242	29.0	± 3.4	20.9	36.0
> 25 ... ≤ 30	25.8	43	33.3	± 0.5	32.0	34.3
SD = standard deviation		3519				

Discussion

During the first twelve months of the investigation there were nearly no sick boars with increased body temperature. So, vaccination of boars against influenza was used to check the function of QSS 2000 as a warning system, in the expectation of rising body temperature in several boars soon after vaccination. Indeed, 38 % of the boars showed a rectal temperature of 39.3 °C or more in the first six hours after vaccination. But the coefficient of correlation with the skin temperature at the ear was low (r = 0.31). Possible reasons for that are the influence of room temperature on ear temperature and the diurnal rhythm of ear temperature, with the lowest temperature accompanied with the highest standard deviation in the early morning and the peak, together with the lowest standard deviation in the afternoon.

Conclusions

It seems to be impossible to define a fixed upper bound of warning temperature. This corresponds with results from Zinn et al. (1985), who found that the correlation of skin and rectal temperature was low (mean r^2 from 0.007 to 0.273). In future work the definition of a flexible corridor calculated under consideration of the individual diurnal curve of ear temperature for each boar and the different variations during night and day to be used as an early warning tool will be developed. This curve should represent the means per hour ± standard deviation.

References

Roehlinger, P., Guenther, M., Danz, J., Lyhs, L. and Zimmerhackel, M. 1979. Zur Anwendung der Infrarottechnik in der Veterinärmedizin. (Application of infrared technique in veterinary medicine). Arch. exper. Vet. med. 33 (6), 851-856

Roehlinger, P., Grunow, Ch. and Börnert, D. 1980. Ergebnisse berühungsloser Messung der Oberflächentemperatur beim Schwein.(Results of contactless surface temperature measurement in swine). Arch. exper. Vet. med. 34 (5), 759-766

Zinn, K.R., Zinn, G.M., Jesse, G.W., Mayes, H.F. and Ellersieck, M.R. 1985. Correlation of noninvasive surface temperature measurements with rectal temperature in swine. Am. J. Vet. Res. 46 (6), 1372-1374

Acknowledgement

This project was funded by the Federal Ministry of Economics and Technoloy.

Controlling growth of broiler chickens on-line, based on a compact predictive growth model

D. Berckmans, J.-M. Aerts and S. Van Buggenhout
Laboratory for Agricultural Building Research, Department of Agro-engineering and -Economics, Catholic University of Leuven, Kasteelpark Arenberg 30, B-3001 Leuven, Belgium
Daniel.berckmans@agr.kuleuven.ac.be

Abstract

It was aimed to develop a model-based control algorithm that allows control of the growth trajectory of broiler chickens by control of their food supply. In order to develop the control algorithm, 'Model Predictive Control' theory (MPC) was applied. Two experiments were conducted on a small scale (50 animals) and three experiments were carried out on a large scale (2900 animals). To test the usefulness of the model-based control algorithm, different target trajectories were defined ranging from severe restricted growth trajectories to pronounced compensatory growth trajectories. The control algorithm managed to realise the predefined reference trajectory with a Mean Relative Error (MRE) that varied between 3.7% and 5.3%.

Keywords: broiler chickens, growth, model-based control, recursive parameter estimation

Introduction

Genetic selection and improved nutrition have led to a reduction of the commercial slaughter age in broiler chickens. This evolution has resulted in several negative growth responses (Plavnik et al., 1986; Lippens et al., 2000). These negative growth responses can be reduced by altering the growth trajectory in such a way that the initial growth is lowered, followed by an accelerated growth, i.e. compensatory growth (Auckland and Morris, 1971; Zubair & Leeson, 1996).

To control the growth trajectory during the growth process, food supply has proved to be one of the most important process inputs which can be used. Economically, food is also an important input since it accounts for more than 70 % of total broiler production costs (Filmer, 2000). One way to control processes, such as growth processes, in a more optimal way is by applying model-based control theory (Camacho & Bordons, 1999). Such control strategies require the availability of a process model that allows predicting the dynamic response of the process output to the control input. For implementation in practice, such models should be as compact and accurate as possible. This research was aimed at developing a model-based control algorithm that allows controlling the growth trajectory of broiler chickens by means of the control input food supply.

Materials and methods

Model-based growth control

In the reported research, it was assumed that the relation between cumulative feed intake and weight, which is non-linear (Brody, 1945; Fitzhugh, 1976; Parks, 1982), could be described by recursive linear relations between both variables. So, on each discrete time instant k, the following linear relation can be written:

$$W_k = \theta_{1k} + \theta_{2k} \cdot CF_k \tag{1}$$

where W_k is the measured weight (kg) of the animals at time k; CF_k is the measured cumulative feed intake in kg at time k; θ_{1k} (kg) and θ_{2k} (kg/kg) are the model parameters estimated at time k (days). The parameters were estimated daily, based on a time window of five days. For a more detailed description, the reader is referred to the work of Aerts et al. (2003).

In order to develop the control algorithm, 'Model Predictive Control' theory (MPC) was used. In general, it tries to predict and to control the future process output in such a way that it follows a previously defined target trajectory and at the same time minimises the control effort necessary to follow this target trajectory. This can be achieved by minimising an object function (Camacho & Bordons, 1999). In this research, the object function J was described as:

$$ J(N_1, N_2, N_u) = \sum_{F=N_1}^{N_2} \delta \left[\hat{W}_{k+F|k} - r_{k+F} \right]^2 + \sum_{F=1}^{N_u} \lambda \left[\Delta CF_{k+F-1} \right]^2 \tag{2} $$

with $\hat{W}_{k+F|k}$ the predicted weight of the animals; CF the cumulative food supply; r the reference or target weight trajectory; δ, λ are weighing coefficients; N_1 the minimum cost horizon (set to 1 day in this application); N_2 the maximum cost horizon (set to 4 days in this application); N_u is the control horizon (set to 4 days in this application). After calculation of the optimal sequence of the control input over the control horizon (4 days in this case), only the first value of the calculated control input is applied; then the window is moved with one measuring unit (1 day) and subsequently the procedure of optimisation is repeated with new measured information (i.e. receding horizon principle).

Experiments

In order to test the model-based control of the growth of broiler chicken, five (two small scale and three large scale) experiments were carried out.

Small scale experiments
Birds and Housing: Two experiments (EXP2001-2, 3) were conducted with mixed sex Ross 308 broilers obtained from a local hatchery. The female broiler breeder parent stock was aged 45 weeks. Birds were kept in two climate-controlled rooms each with 4 pens of 50 birds with a stocking density of 16 birds /m². Each pen was equipped with an automatic weighing system for continuous measurement of weight. The average weight of the group was calculated every 24 hours. Total weight of food consumed for each pen was recorded daily (accuracy ± 20g).

Diets: In the two rooms, broilers were fed on a two stage feeding program. A starter diet with 22.1 % CP and 12.1 MJ AME/kg was given until 12 days of age. From day 13 until day 42 a grower diet with 20.5 % CP and 12.7 MJ AME/kg was offered.

Experimental Design: A conventional lighting schedule of 23 h of light and 1 h of darkness was used. Mean air temperature was 30° C during the first three days. On day 4, temperature was set at 28°C. It then decreased by 1°C every three days until a constant temperature of 21°C was reached at day 25. One temperature sensor per room was used for temperature control, mounted in the middle of each room at a distance of approximately 2 m above the floor. Water was freely available to all birds. The growth trial was carried out for 42 days. In each experiment there were four reference groups and four controlled groups (each time, two in room 1 and two in room 2). The reference groups were fed *ad libitum*. The amount of food supplied to the controlled groups was calculated with the control algorithm. The food was offered each day at 9 a.m. as one food. In EXP2001-2, a restricted target growth trajectory was defined with a final body weight, BW, of 1800 g and in EXP2001-3 a compensatory target growth trajectory was defined with a final BW of 2400 g.

Large scale experiments
Birds and Housing: Three experiments (GP2009, 2010 and 2011) were conducted with mixed sex Ross 308 broilers obtained from a local hatchery. The female broiler breeder parent stock was aged 45 weeks. Birds were kept in two climate-controlled compartments with 2900 chickens each (stocking density of 16 birds per m^2). Both compartments were in the same stable. Each compartment was equipped with 4 automatic weighing systems for measuring continuously the weight and calculating the average weight of the group animals every 24 hours. The mean coefficient of variation of the weighing systems was 1.3% for experiment GP2009, 1.3 % for experiment GP2010, and 1.2% for experiment GP2011. The total amount of food consumed per compartment was recorded daily with an accuracy of ± 20 g.
Diets: In the two compartments, broilers were fed on a two stage feeding program. The first 10 days a starter diet with 21.0 % CP and 12.4 MJ AME/kg was given. From day 11 until day 42 the birds were fed with a grower diet with 20.5 % CP and 12.7 MJ AME/kg. Water and food were freely available to all birds during the entire trial.
Experimental Design: During the three experiments, classic temperature and lighting schemes were applied in both compartments (cf. idem as small scale experiments). Air temperature was controlled per compartment based on the average temperature, measured by means of two temperature sensors, mounted in the middle of quadrant 1 and 3 at a distance of 0.8 m above the floor. In one compartment, the animals were fed *ad libitum* (reference group) and in the other compartment the food supply was calculated based on the control algorithm (controlled group). Because both compartments were not identical, the controlled group and the *ad libitum* fed group were changed among the compartments during the successive trials. The on-line modelling concept used the mean weight of a group of broilers (calculated each 24 hours) and the mean daily food intake of each section as input. In GP2009 and GP2010, a restricted target growth trajectory was defined (final BW of 1945 g). In GP2011 a compensatory target growth trajectory was defined (final BW of 2014 g). This trajectory was determined based on results of previous experiments with food restrictions performed in the same stable and with the same genetic line of animals.

Results and discussion

In Table 1, an overview of the performance of the control algorithm for all experiments is shown. The performance was quantified by means of the mean relative error (MRE) which was defined as the average value of the daily absolute relative deviations between the measured liveweight and the target reference liveweight (%).

Table 1. Overview of the MRE and mortality for all experiments.

Experiment nr.	Number of animals housed per pen/compartment	Mortality (%)	MRE (%)
EXP2001-2	50	4.6	3.7, 4.1[*]
EXP2001-3	50	2.2	4.6, 5.3[*]
GP2009	2900	3.1	4
GP2010	2900	2.5	3.7
GP2011	2900	4.2	4.8

[*]MRE values per climate-controlled room.

An overview of the measured liveweights, cumulative food consumption, target trajectories and food conversion rates for the *ad libitum* fed animals and the controlled animals of experiments GP2009, GP2010 and GP2011 is given in Table 2.

Table 2. Measured liveweights, cumulative food consumption, target trajectories (Traj.) and food conversion rates for the *ad libitum* fed animals (ad-lib) and the controlled animals (Cont.) of experiments GP2009, GP2010 and GP2011.

Liveweight (mean in g)

Age Days	EXP GP2009			EXP GP2010			EXP GP2011		
	ad-lib	Traj.	Cont.	ad-lib	Traj.	Cont.	ad-lib	Traj.	Cont.
7	137	113	108	117	113	106	120	119	109
14	314	295	274	285	295	278	301	269	273
21	616	555	530	588	555	547	637	560	539
28	1081	886	846	940	886	910	1044	1008	963
35	1462	1226	1236	1365	1226	1349	1519	1542	1428
42	2219	1945	1964	1993	1945	1935	2078	2104	2061

Food intake (g cumulative to date)

Age Days	EXPGP2009		EXPGP2010		EXPGP2011	
	ad-lib	Cont.	ad-lib	Cont.	ad-lib	Cont.
7	112	90	97	110	117	106
14	377	352	416	349	405	354
21	858	772	833	762	926	774
28	1603	1362	1471	1277	1608	1539
35	2592	2390	2333	2083	2597	2485
42	3733	3597	3442	3193	3746	3666

Food conversion to date

Age Days	EXPGP2009		EXPGP2010		EXPGP2011	
	ad-lib	Cont.	ad-lib	Cont.	ad-lib	Cont.
7	1.55	1.29	1.45	1.95	1.67	1.79
14	1.57	1.42	1.77	1.53	1.61	1.59
21	1.60	1.52	1.55	1.53	1.60	1.58
28	1.71	1.55	1.65	1.48	1.61	1.68
35	2.01	1.84	1.77	1.60	1.77	1.80
42	1.88	1.72	1.77	1.69	1.84	1.82

In order to test the model-based control algorithm, different reference trajectories were used. During experiment EXP2001-2, the animals were restricted during the whole growing period (BW of 1800 g on day 42). In experiment EXP2001-3, a pronounced compensatory growth trajectory was followed (BW of 2400 g on day 42). In experiment EXP2001-2, the animals in both rooms were able to realize the reference growth trajectory. The *MRE* was 3.7% in the first room and 4.1% in the second room. In experiment EXP2001-3 a growth trajectory with strong compensatory growth (initial lowered growth followed by an accelerated growth) was applied. In both climate-controlled rooms, the model-based control algorithm was able to follow the reference trajectory (for an example, see figure 1). In room 2, the controlled group realized a complete compensatory growth in comparison with the reference animals (fed *ad libitum*). The *MRE* was 4.6% in room 1 and 5.3% in room 2. A graphical result of model-based growth control for the small-scale experiments (50 animals) is presented in figure 1. In this figure the controlled trajectory, the reference trajectory, the trajectory of the *ad libitum* group and also the relative error (%) were drawn as functions of time.

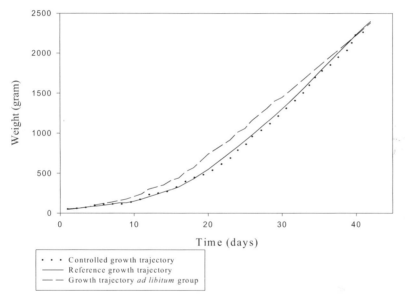

Figure 1. Path of the controlled growth trajectory, reference trajectory, the growth trajectory of the reference group in function of time (EXP2001-3, room 2, 50 animals).

In experiments GP2009 and GP2010, a moderate restricted growth trajectory (a final BW of 1945 g), was set as reference. In experiment GP 2011, a more realistic growth trajectory (final BW of 2104 g) was set as reference. The birds were able to follow up the previously defined target growth trajectory with a mean relative error (cf. eq. 3) smaller than 5% (MRE of 4% in GP2009, a MRE of 3.7% in GP2010 and a MRE of 4.8% in GP2011).

Although one might expect that dominant birds eat more of their fair share of food during food restrictions than recessive birds, this was not observed in terms of uniformity of liveweight in the controlled groups compared to the reference groups. The uniformity index, calculated as the percentage of birds that were within 10% of the mean BW of all the birds of the group, of the controlled birds compared to reference (*ad libitum* fed) birds was 57% vs. 40% (GP2009), 47% vs. 55% (GP2010) and 56% vs. 50% (GP2011).

Conclusions

In this research it is demonstrated that the principle of combining on-line measured weight of broilers during the growth process with compact dynamic data-based models could be used to control growth trajectories by applying modern control theory. The developed control algorithm was able to grow the birds according to different target trajectories ranging from severely restricted (final BW of 1800 g) to pronounced compensatory growth trajectories (final BW of 2400 g). The mean relative error (MRE) between the previously target growth trajectories and the realized growth trajectories ranged from 3.7% up to 5.3%. Further testing is needed in field conditions since in this research experiments were performed only on small groups of animals (50 and 2900 birds) and with low stocking densities (16 birds/m^2). An important control input that could be included in future is food composition. It can be stated that the integration of dynamic data-based modelling approaches with new hardware techniques and sensors and/or sensing techniques, should make it possible to model animal responses (the most important process part) to variations of process control inputs. This is a basis for advanced model predictive control of bioprocesses.

The fact that biological systems are much more complex than mechanical systems, makes the process control more challenging.

References

Aerts J.-M., Lippens M., De Groote G., Buyse J., Decuypere E., Vranken E., Berckmans D. 2003. Recursive Prediction of Broiler Growth Response to feed intake by using a Time-variant Parameter Estimation Method. Poultry Science 82(1): 40-49.

Auckland, J. N., and T. R. Morris, 1971. Compensatory growth in turkeys: effect of under-nutrition on subsequent protein requirements. British Poultry Science, 12: 41-48.

Brody, S., 1945. Bioenergetics and growth. With special reference to the efficiency complex in domestic animals. New York, Reinhold.

Camacho E. F. and C. Bordons. 1999. Model predictive control. Springer-Verlag, Berlin.

Filmer, D. 2000. Nutritional management of meat poultry. In: Integrated management systems for livestock, Occasional Publication No 28. British Society of Animal Science: 133-146.

Fitzhugh, H. A., 1976. Analysis of growth curves and strategies for altering shape. Journal of Animal Science, 42: 1036-1051.

Lippens M., Room G., De Groote G., Decuypere E. 2000. Early and temporary quantitative food restriction of broiler chickens. 1. Effects on performance characteristics, mortality and meat quality. British Poultry Science, 41: 343-354.

Parks, J. R., 1982. A theory of feeding and growth of animals., Springer-Verlag, Berlin.

Plavnik, I., McMurtry, J. P., and R. W. Rosebrough, 1986. Effect of early food restriction in broilers. I. Growth performance and carcass composition. Growth, 50: 68-76.

Zubair, A. K., and S. Leeson, 1996. Compensatory growth in the broiler chickens: a review. World's Poultry Science Journal, 52: 189-201.

Acknowledgements

We wish to thank the Belgian Ministry of Small Enterprises and Agriculture - Research and Development and Fancom b.v. for funding this research.

Non-invasive sensors for monitoring the body temperature and heart rate of pigs during transport

E.D. Chesmore[1], C.S. Yoon[1], J.C. Talling[2], K.S. Van Driel[2] and M. Lake[3]
[1]Department of Electronics, University of York, York, YO10 5DD, UK
[2]Central Science Laboratory, Sand Hutton, York, YO41 1LZ, UK
[3]Pig Unit Manager, Bishop Burton College, Bishop Burton, Beverley, HU17 8QD, UK
edc1@york.ac.uk

Abstract

A miniature non-invasive biotelemetry system has been designed that is capable of transmitting via radio body temperature and heart rate of pigs during transport. The sensors are placed within the animal's ear canal and the system is capable of monitoring up to 32 animals simultaneously using a single licence exempt radio channel. The paper describes the development of the system and results of experimental trials conducted on pigs under commercial conditions. The system can also receive data from custom-designed battery-powered environmental sensor units deployed at various points within a vehicle.

Keywords: pigs, biotelemetry systems, stress monitoring, animal welfare, animal transport.

Introduction

The transport of farm animals can induce severe stress but relatively little is known about the relationship between aspects of the transport environment and the stress response. One of the major reasons for this has been the lack of reliable non-invasive techniques that can be used to monitor stress under normal commercial conditions. Immunological measurements are most helpful for assessing chronic stress, such as that caused by housing, whilst hormones and physical factors, such as heart rate, are more important for assessing acute stress. Heat stress is a great hazard when transporting animals; particularly to animals like pigs who cannot sweat but rely upon behavioural responses to lose heat (e.g. wallowing in mud) that cannot be performed inside a lorry. Until now, it has been difficult to measure physiological stress in pigs during transport because of the lack of available sensors (von Borell, 2001). Those that are available are either invasive, requiring surgery, or are attached using belts that are frequently removed by the pig. This paper describes an alternative non-invasive approach using sensors placed within the animal's ear which provides a high level of immunity to interference from the animal itself and conspecifics (Talling, 2002). The sensor is fixed within the animal's ear by soft expandable foam similar to that used for human ear defenders and by prosthetic glue. An additional advantage of using the foam is that it provides a good seal around the ear thus minimising any cooling effects from the environment. Each ear sensor has a temperature sensor and heart rate sensor connected to a microcontroller and a 433MHz licence exempt low power radio transmitter. A simple time division multiplexing technique has been designed to enable up to 32 sensors to operate nearly simultaneously over the same channel. Data from all sensors is received by a single radio receiver and collected by a portable computer. In addition to the ear sensors, the system can receive data from a number of battery powered environmental sensor units which can be placed at suitable locations within the vehicle. Each environmental sensor unit currently measures temperature and relative humidity but the range of sensors can easily be expanded to include vibration, sound pressure level, etc. A summary of the sensor system's specifications are given in Table 1. Prior to implementation of the sensor, tests were carried out to determine the behavioural response of pigs to the insertion of a biotelemetry implant.

Mock-ups of implants were made from expanding foam and fixed into the ears of 8 pigs with prosthetic glue; 8 control pigs were handled in a similar manner but without the implant being inserted. The implants stayed in the ears for a mean of 3 days with a range of 24 hours to 7 days. The only response of the pigs to the implant was head shaking with a mean number of shakes in 1 hour of 13.3 (s.e. ±4.5) and a range of 7 to 24 (Inglis, 2000; Talling et al, 2002). The head shaking showed a significant decrease over time.

Table 1. Specifications of the non-invasive sensor system.

Ear sensor unit

Temperature range and resolution	29.3°C to 42.05°C, 0.05°C resolution
Heart rate range and resolution	0-255 beats per minute, single beat resolution
Transmission range	7m indoors
Operating life (silver oxide cell 16mAh)	8 days at 10 minute transmission interval

Environmental sensor unit

Temperature range and resolution	-40°C to 87.5•C, 0.5°C resolution
Relative humidity range and resolution	10% RH to 100% RH, 1% RH resolution
Transmission range	>20m (theoretically up to 75m in open field)
Operating life (AA alkaline cells, 2700mAh)	53 days

Ear sensor

The ear sensor is shown in Photograph 1 and consists of a step-up power converter, a microcontroller, radio transmitter, temperature sensor and heart rate sensor. The microcontroller (Microchip Inc PIC series) performs all sampling and manipulation of sensor values and transmission of the data. Temperature is measured with a commercial temperature sensor integrated circuit whose output is 10mV°C^{-1}. The output is scaled to give a range of 29.3°C to 42.05°C and sampled by the microcontroller's internal analogue to digital converter. Heart rate is measured by monitoring fluctuations in light from an LED caused by blood flow in the ear's blood vessels. The microcontroller actively controls the LED output and light intensity is measured with

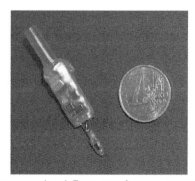

Photograph 1. Ear sensor shown with a 1 Euro coin for size comparison.

a photodiode. Data is transmitted at approximately 10 minute intervals at 600 bits/second to the receiver via a 433MHz licence exempt radio telemetry transmitter using a helical antenna to ensure a small physical size.

One of the novel features of the system is that only transmitters are used due to size considerations. With transmission only, it is possible for more than one sensor to transmit at the same time, resulting in interference (a 'collision') that the receiver cannot resolve, i.e. loss of data. The transmission protocol is based on a time division multiple access (TDMA) approach where each transmitter has a time interval in which to transmit. Collisions are reduced by adding a random time delay before transmission so that the likelihood of two or more simultaneous transmissions is reduced considerably. Longer intervals between transmission with further reduce the likelihood of collision. Power consumption is of paramount importance in the ear sensor and the microcontroller actively controls power to the sensors and transmitter to minimise consumption. The sensor is powered by a single silver oxide cell and an operating life of 8 days has been achieved with a transmission interval of 10 minutes. The operating life can be extended by increasing the interval. Transmission distance is dependent on the physical environment in which the pig is placed. A large amount of metal can reduce transmission distance. Typical distances of 7m have been obtained in the trials which are suitable for use within the transport environment.

Environmental sensor design

The environmental sensor unit is designed along similar lines as the ear sensor but size is not a limitation. Hence, power can be supplied by a larger capacity cell, resulting in a much longer operational lifetime, typically over 50 days with a 2700mAh cell. The temperature range is -40°C to 87.5°C with 0.5°C resolution to encompass the likely range of temperatures encountered within a transport vehicle. Relative humidity is measured with a resistive humidity sensing module with a range of 10% RH to 100% RH at 1% RH resolution. Data is transmitted at 600 bits/second with a 16-bit CRC checksum using TDMA in an identical manner to the ear sensor. The larger size of the unit allows a full size whip antenna to be used, giving a much longer transmission distance of 20m with up to 75m in an open uncluttered environment.

Radio receiver and data logger

Photograph 2 shows the radio receiver, environmental and ear sensors and the data logging software. The radio receiver is connected to a portable PC via the serial port configured to 600 baud. Data logging software, written in Microsoft Visual BASIC v6.0 running under Windows ME, performs all data packet identification, CRC checking, display and data logging. In the final version, the portable PC will be replaced by a rugged cabin mounted computer.

Trial results and discussion

Testing of the sensors involved the use of 21 adult sows and 2 small gilts housed under commercial conditions within the pig unit at Bishop Burton College, and also 2 experimental pigs placed within temperature-controlled rooms at the Roslin Institute. It was found that pigs did not need to be restrained during the sensor insertion process; it was simply necessary to distract them with a toy or food. The insertion procedure involved cleaning the ear with cotton wool and surgical spirit, wrapping the sensor in the foam, putting prosthetic glue on the foam and the ear, squeezing the foam and pushing it into the ear as far as possible whilst keeping the pig distracted. Extensive testing was carried out both at Roslin Institute in environmental chambers and in the commercial pig unit at Bishop Burton College. Figure 1 shows temperature data from a sensor in the ear of a small gilt housed singly within a pen at Bishop Burton College over a 2 hour period. It is evident

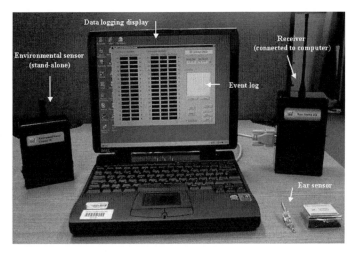

Photograph 2. Receiver PC and data logger software.

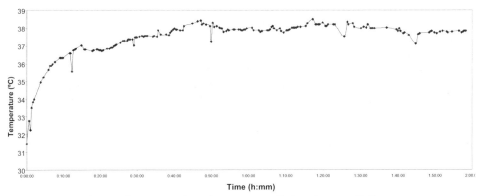

Figure 1. Results for small gilt housed singly in a pen at Bishop Burton College.

that the sensor takes time to reach equilibrium, in this case around 40 minutes. The short duration drops in temperature are caused by the pig the pig shaking its head.

Figure 2 shows 5 hours of data from the ear of an adult sow at Bishop Burton College. In this case, the temperature stabilised after approximately 20 minutes. The graph also shows transients caused by head shakes, the sensor falling out and being replaced and a 25 minute loss of communication when the animal laid down with the ear containing the sensor on the ground. The pig's body temperature was also measured at intervals using a vaginal probe. The sensor has also been tested in an environmental chamber at Roslin Institute on a pig with an implanted biotelemetry sensor in the abdominal body cavity. In a hot room test (31°C, 65% RH and 2ms^{-1} wind speed) the ear sensor stabilised at 0.4°C below the body cavity temperature. In a cold test (-1°C, 55% RH and 2ms^{-1} wind speed), the ear sensor stabilised at 1°C below that of the body cavity; a vaginal reading showed a higher temperature than the ear but lower than the body cavity. Under cold and windy conditions, the ear temperature dropped significantly indicating a poor seal in the ear.

Multi-channel operation has also been tested on 16 pigs in pens at Bishop Burton College. Data has not been presented here due to lack of space. The heart rate sensor is still under development

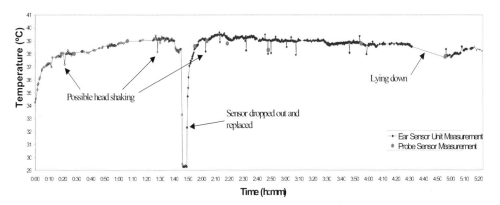

Figure 2. Sensor data from an adult sow housed singly at Bishop Burton College.

- preliminary trials show that the sensor is more sensitive to head movements than the temperature sensor and investigations are under way to improve the sensor reliability.

Conclusions

Monitoring of stress in animals during transport has previously been difficult to achieve and expensive. The system described here provides near simultaneous monitoring of body temperature from up to 32 animals in a non-invasive manner. Ear sensors are low cost and can be applied easily. Body temperature measured in the ear closely follows vaginal temperature under normal conditions but is lower under windy conditions, possibly due to heat loss through the foam insert. Heart rate has been tested but not implemented in the current version. Future developments include further reduction in physical size of the ear sensor through recently developed microcontrollers with embedded radio transmitters and improvement in the foam seal.

References

Inglis, I. 2000. To assess the behavioural responses of pigs to a biotelemetry sensor placed in the ear canal. DEFRA Project Number AW0811.

Talling, J.C. 2002. Non-invasive sensor to monitor the body temperature and heart rate of pigs. DEFRA project no AW0814.

Talling, J.C., van Driel, K.S., Yoon, D.C., Chesmore, D., Inglis, I.R. and Lake, M. 2002. Development of an ear sensor to measure body temperature and heart rate in pigs. Proceedings of the 36th International Congress of the ISAE, 61.

von Borell, E.H. 2001. The biology of stress and its application to livestock housing and transportation assessment. Journal of Animal Science 79 260-267.

Acknowledgements

The project was funded by the Department of Environment, Food and Rural Affairs (DEFRA), project nos. AW0811 and AW0814.

A proposed new empirical model for the lactation curve of the cow and its use with a milking database for farm management

G.C. Di Renzo[1], G. Altieri[1], G. Giuratrabocchetti[2] and A.Colangelo[2]
[1]*University of Basilicata, I-85100, Potenza, Italy*
[2]*Associazione Provinciale Allevatori-Potenza, I-85100, Potenza, Italy*
Altieri@unibas.it

Abstract

On a dairy cattle farm in Basilicata over a three-year period, for cows milked twice per day, milking data were collected using an automatic system based on electronic individual identification of cows and their related milk yields. Using collected data a new empirical model of the cow lactation curve was tested in order to verify its predictive capacity in comparison with other existing models.

The model proposed uses the cubic b-spline function as an approximating function on 6 variable knots sequence. The models considered were: spline3-6 (6 variable knots), spline3-5 (5 variable knots), lognormal4 (a general peak approximating function), Guo95, Wilmink87, Ali87, Emmans86, Wood67, Nelder66, Brody45. The cubic b-spline with 6 variable knots achieved the best score (S).

A possible use of the model with respect to the lactation curve database involves the definition of the "mean productivity index after 305 days from calving" (IPM305): this is defined as the average value of the lactation curve over the specified 305-day period. Two useful guideline applications are proposed and discussed: the first involves the positioning of the daily milk yield onto the herd lactation curve model; the second concerns the comparison of IPM305 of each cow with respect to the IPM305 of the herd averaged over all the cows (HIPM305).

Keywords: cow, farm, management, model, lactation curve.

Introduction

Successful dairy farm management usually involves the strict observation of health regulations and careful genetic selection of cows, which are considered the first steps to increase the farm production level in terms of quality and quantity.

In order to improve farm management, genetic analysis, trait selection and nutritional decisions, exact knowledge of milk traits and milk yield is required. Furthermore, the traits with low relative daily variation (such as lactose and protein content) need to be recorded less frequently than the traits with high daily variation (such as milk yield and fat content) that need to be recorded daily (Svennersten-Sjaunja et al., 1997; Rekaya et al., 1999). This requires the ability to rapidly and reliably identify each cow in the herd, and then combining the individual cow code with the cow milking data.

This fundamental step would not have been possible without the application of electronics for sensors, control units and on-line monitoring devices. Such devices permit the data monitoring of the traits of each individual milking operation that may be useful in giving forewarning of cow disorders (Ordolff, 2001; Artmann, 1999). For example, by using an in-line measurement in the near infrared spectrum it is possible achieve a reliable count of somatic cells in milk during the milking operation (Pravdova et al., 2001). Thus the farmer may have the necessary tools to control herd production and monitor the health status of each cow.

A mathematical or empirical model of the cow lactation curve provides information that is useful for management and breeding decisions. This objective is achieved when daily milk yield may be predicted with minimum error. Thus the milk production pattern may be monitored even in the presence of high environmental variation (Olori et. al., 1999).

The usefulness of any empirical or mathematical model relies on how well it can predict the trend in the lactation curve. So as to improve the existing prediction model for the cow lactation curve, a new empirical model was constructed.

Materials and methods

The data used in this work were obtained from an automatic collection system in a herd on the Ferramosca farm situated in Basilicata (Southern Italy) with about 50 Bruna Alpina cows in lactation over a period of three years. Cows were milked twice per day and milking data were collected using a TDM-Afikim automatic system based on electronic individual identification of cows using a Gesympex ruminal bolus containing a transponder; relative milk yields were measured using an Afikim MM95 electronic milk flowmeter. This constituted the milking-database that was formed by: cow individual code, day and time of milking, daily milk production, milking maximum flow peak.

The cows were individually identified automatically by the following procedure: the animal goes through a portal-like radio antenna that triggers the transponder contained in the ruminal bolus inside the reticulum of the cow. First the electric field of the antenna irradiates the cow, charging the internal battery of the bolus; then the bolus emits its own unique identifying code that is received by the antenna itself. A so-called "collector" electronic device then combines the unique code of the cow with the milking data recorded by the flowmeter. On a regular basis the personal computer holding the milking-database transmitted the new collected records to the farmers association (APA-PZ) for their storage. For data analysis, use was made of a commercial software program commonly applied for statistical data analysis called TableCurve™2D version 5 (© 2000 AISN Software Inc., P.O. Box 449, Mapleton, OR 97453).

Mathematical models for the cow lactation curve

To use the cow lactation curve for statistical purposes in order to control and improve farm production it is necessary to build empirical or mathematical models that allow the mean lactation curve of the farm to be obtained in relation to each cow and even to its number of parities; this allows each cow's lactation curve to be compared with the farm mean lactation curve for the prediction of stressed cows. This comparison can help the farm manager to perform genetic analysis and trait selection, which makes the model more suitable for use in farm management software.

The models used to this aim are empirical or mechanistic (Cappio-Borlino et al., 1997; Pulina et al., 2001; Olori et al., 1999; Friggens et al., 1999; Garcia and Holmes, 2001; Pool and Meuwissen, 2000; Rekaya et al., 2001) or based on a mixed neuro-fuzzy logic (Salehi et al., 2000).

The models considered are: the Brody model (1945) (BRODY45); the Nelder model (1966) (NELDER66); the Wood model (1967) (WOOD67); the Emmans model (1986) (EMMANS86); the Ali model (1987) (ALI87); the Wilmink model (1987) (WILMINK87); the Guo model (1995) (GUO95).

WOOD67, NELDER66, WILMINK87, GUO95 and ALI87 as reported in Olori et al., 1999; EMMANS86 as reported in Friggens et al., 1999; BRODY45 as reported in Pulina et al., 2001 and Cappio-Borlino et al., 1997.

Moreover the following empirical models proposed by the authors will be considered: model by LogNormal curve with 4 parameters (LOGNORMAL4); model by cubic b-spline with 5 variable knots (B-SPLINE 3-5); model by cubic b-spline with 6 variable knots (B-SPLINE 3-6).

Furthermore the multiphasic model of Grossman & Koops, 1988, as reported in Garcia & Holmes, 2001, has not been considered as it seems unsuitable for the milking data obtained from these cows in lactation.

Mathematical equations of models under evaluation

In the following equations y(t) is the mean daily milk yield at day t, while "a", "b", "c", "d" and "e" are parameters that shape the lactation curve, Y0 is an offset parameter.

The equations of models under evaluation are: **BRODY45 model:** $y(t)=a \cdot \exp(-b \cdot t)+c \cdot \exp(-d \cdot t)$; **NELDER66 model:** $y(t)=t \cdot (a+b \cdot t+ c \cdot t^2)^{-1}$; **WOOD67 model:** $y(t)=a \cdot t^b \cdot \exp(-c \cdot t)$; **EMMANS86 model:** $y(t)=a \cdot \{\exp[-\exp(d-b(t)]\} \cdot \exp(-d \cdot t)$; **ALI87 model:** $y(t)=a+b \cdot t+c \cdot t^2+d \cdot \ln(t)+e \cdot \ln^2(t)$; **WILMINK87 model:** $y(t)=a+b \cdot \exp(-c \cdot t)+d \cdot t$; **GUO95 model:** $y(t)=a+b \cdot t^{(1/2)}+c \cdot \ln(t)$; **LOGNORMAL4 model:** $y(t)=Y0+a \cdot \exp[-\ln(2)/\ln(d)^2 \cdot \ln[(t-b) \cdot (d^2-1)/(c \cdot d)+1]^2]$; **Models with cubic B-SPLINES (Basic splines) with variable knots:** this empirical model is proposed by the authors and is based upon the use of the cubic b-splines function as an approximating function (via the least squares criterion) on a 5 or 6 variable knots sequence; such a function, and more generally piecewise polynomial functions, is used to successfully approximate experimental data or design curve measurements. Such functions are commonly used in engineering when curves interpolating experimental data are required that have a polynomial equation and are extremely smoothed. (De Boor, 1968; De Boor & Rice, 1968a; De Boor & Rice, 1968b; De Boor, 1976; De Boor, 1981). For the empirical model of the cow lactation curve the authors suggest the use of cubic b-splines using 5 or 6 variable knots (B-SPLINE 3-5 model and B-SPLINE 3-6 model).

Best fit evaluation of the empirical models when applied to the experimental data

The parameters used to test the best fit of models to the milking data were: the squared correlation coefficient R^2 (R2) and the standard error (SE) both on the overall data population of the lactation curve (R2c and SEc) and on the mean lactation curve (R2m and SEm). Moreover, on the mean lactation curve the sum of the absolute value of the relative error (SSR) was considered as an indicator of the global error between the mathematical equation of the model and the mean lactation curve (Snedecor & Coochran, 1989). These coefficients were then normalised to obtain a value in the range from 0 to 1 as follows: NR2=(R2-R2min)/(R2max-R2min); in this equation R2min and R2max are respectively the minimum and maximum value derived from all considered models, R2 is the value from the current model and NR2 is the obtained normalised value for the current model.

For standard error the normalisation procedure is exactly the same but reversed, in the sense that a high standard error is normalised toward 0 while a low standard error is normalised toward 1. This is obtained as follows: NSE=(SEmax-SE)/(SEmax-SEmin). The same normalisation is applied to the SSR, the equation being: NSSR=(SSRmax-SSR)/(SSRmax-SSRmin).

After coefficient normalisation a function was constructed that acted as a score (S) for each model. This score S is high when the fit of the model to experimental data is high. Such a function is simply an arithmetic mean with equal weights of the five previously considered coefficients that were selected as indicators of good fit.

In this manner the score S is a value ranging from 0 to 1 obtained as follows: S=(NR2c+NSEc+NR2m+NSEm+NSSR)/5.

Results and discussion

Table 1 lists the scores S for each model with respect to the number of parities of the cows, while Table 2 lists the ranking in descending order of scores of each model for cows with one, two and three or more parities.

From Table 2 it emerges that the model that best fits the experimental data of milk yield is B-SPLINE 3-6. Thus this model will be used on subsequent analysis of milk yield.

From the previous tables analysis it may be inferred that the B-SPLINE 3-6 model supersedes every other model in terms of the best fit of the experimental data. Moreover, for cows with two or three or more parities the ALI-87 model achieved the second highest score S. The LOGNORMAL4 model, a general peak approximating function, does not give the expected good results.

Table 1. Scores S for each model when applied to the experimental data for cows with one, two and three or more parities.

"Bruna Alpina"	Score S		
	One parity	Two parities	Three or more parities
BRODY45	0.68	0.33	0.43
NELDER66	0.33	0.15	0.18
WOOD67	0.20	0.44	0.80
EMMANS86	0.66	0.25	0.36
ALI87	0.60	0.84	0.90
WILMINK87	0.70	0.59	0.56
GUO95	0.63	0.83	0.81
LOGNORMAL4	0.70	0.62	0.69
B-SPLINE 3-5	0.68	0.77	0.76
B-SPLINE 3-6	0.86	0.91	0.93

Table 2. Ranking by descending score S for each model when applied to the experimental data for cows with one, two and three or more parities.

Order by diminishing score S		
One parity	Two parities	Three or more parities
B-SPLINE 3-6	B-SPLINE 3-6	B-SPLINE 3-6
WILMINK87	ALI87	ALI87
LOGNORMAL4	GUO95	GUO95
BRODY45	B-SPLINE 3-5	WOOD67
B-SPLINE 3-5	LOGNORMAL4	B-SPLINE 3-5
EMMANS86	WILMINK87	LOGNORMAL4
GUO95	WOOD67	WILMINK87
ALI87	BRODY45	BRODY45
NELDER66	EMMANS86	EMMANS86
WOOD67	NELDER66	NELDER66

The B-SPLINE 3-6 model achieved a great improvement over the other model for cows with one or two parities, with a large gap between the first and second ranked, while for cows with three or more parities the score S reached is very close to those of well established models such as ALI87. Furthermore the B-SPLINE 3-6 model has a score of only 0.86 for cows with one parity: this, also considering the score of the other models, confirm the fact that the fit of the milking data for these cows is very difficult.

The mean productivity index after 305 days from calving (IPM_{305}) as a comparison of productivities

In order to compare lactation curves that are so variable with days after calving, in this work the mean productivity index was defined after 305 days from calving (IPM_{305}). IPM_{305} is the cow lactation curve averaged on 305 days from calving. Hence it is also possible to define a mean productivity index for the herd ($HIPM_{305}$) from the herd mean lactation curve averaged over 305 days. Table 3 lists the values of $HIPM_{305}$, maximum peaks of daily yield and days from calving of this maximum peak both for the mean lactation curve and for the B-SPLINE 3-6 model; from this data it emerges that for the overall of the listed parameters exists a good agreement between the model and the data as obtained from the mean lactation curve of the herd.

Using the mean productivity index, comparisons may be made between two similar herds and between a single cow with respect to the herd. This application is shown in Table 4 where the IPM305 of "Diana" and "Ketty" are compared to the HIPM305 of the herd. Moreover, for this particular case, it must take into account that "Diana" has had three parities while "Ketty" has had 7 parities.

Table 3. $HIPM_{305}$, maximum peak of daily yield and the days from calving of the maximum peak arising for the mean lactation curve and for the B-SPLINE 3-6 model for cows with one, two and three or more parities.

"Bruna Alpina"	Mean lactation curve			B-SPLINE 3-6 model		
	One parity	Two parities	Three or more parities	One parity	Two parities	Three or more parities
$HIPM_{305}$ (l/d)	26.909	26.773	30.064	26.924	26.778	30.063
Max peak (l)	30.356	33.957	36.424	29.797	32.137	35.399
Day of max peak (d)	59	33	59	50	35	53

Table 4. Comparison between the $HIPM_{305}$ and the IPM_{305} of "Diana" and "Ketty".

"Bruna Alpina"	Three or more parities (B-SPLINE 3-6 model)		
	Herd	"Diana" (three parities)	"Ketty" (7 parities)
$HIPM_{305}$ or IPM_{305} (l/d)	30.063	28.918	31.369

The use of the model lactation curve as an early warning system for cow health

In Figure 1 a possible application of the lactation curve is shown as derived from the model. In this case two alarm bands are tuned for the model lactation curve, e.g. in cooperation with the veterinarian. Then the daily milk production of the cow is compared with the curve in question. Positioning outside the lower band may then trigger a warning that may indicate possible health problems for the cow; on the right side of Figure 1 are draft the B-SPLINE 3-6 model for "Diana" and "Ketty" compared with the lactation curve B-SPLINE 3-6 model of the herd.

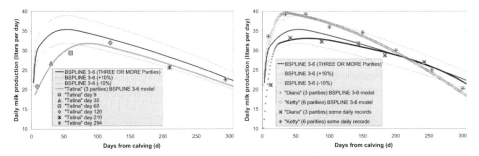

Figure 1. Daily milk production of "Tatina" (3 parities) compared with the lactation curve of the B-SPLINE 3-6 model for cow with three or more parities (on the left side), furthermore (on the right side) the B-SPLINE 3-6 model for "Diana" (3 parities) and "Ketty" (6 parities) that are included in the alarm bands of the herd lactation curve of the B-SPLINE 3-6 model for cow with three or more parities.

Conclusions

From this work it emerges that in order to improve the statistical reliability of the lactation curve model a huge body of data is required and this is solely possible when automatic collection systems are used. Fortunately, electronic science and information technology have permitted the construction of data collection systems with near-zero maintenance.

Data analysis confirmed that the empirical model using the cubic b-splines with 6 variable knots attained the best score when compared with other well-established models. The traits of the cow lactation curve are well depicted by the proposed model, including the lactation peak and the trend to dry off.

The calculated herd lactation curve is a valuable tool for the farm manager, supplying health signals and providing information for genetic analysis. On positioning the daily milk yield onto the herd lactation curve model, a milk yield below the alarm bands (e.g. +/- 10%) with respect to the herd lactation curve model can predict a stressed cow if such bands are well tuned in cooperation with the veterinarian. Furthermore, comparison of IPM305 of each cow with respect to the IPM305 of the herd averaged over all the cows (HIPM305) may assist the farm manager in genetic analysis and trait selection, considered the first steps to increase and improve farm production, and may also help to increase the production of high quality milk.

All these characteristics make the use of a reliable empirical model more suitable for use in software for successful dairy farm management.

Further researches will be run with the aim to verify and compare the herds and to assess the influence of the environmental conditions on the recorded data.

References

Artmann R:, 1999. Electronic identification systems: state of the art and their further development. Computers and Electronics in Agriculture, 24, 5-26.

Cappio-Borlino A., Macciotta N.P.P., Pulina G., 1997. The shape of sarda ewe lactation curve analysed by a compartmental model. Livestock Production Science, 51: 89-96.

De Boor C., 1968. On uniform approximation by splines. J. Approx. Theory 1, 219-235.

De Boor C., Rice J.R., 1968a. Least Squares Cubic Spline Approximation I - Fixed Knots. Department of Computer Sciences Purdue University CSD TR 20.

De Boor C., Rice J.R., 1968b. Least Squares Cubic Spline Approximation II - Variable Knots. Department of Computer Sciences Purdue University CSD TR 21.

De Boor C., 1976. Splines as linear combinations of B-splines. A Survey. in Approximation theory, II, Lorentz G.G., Chui C.K., Schumaker L.L. (ed.), Academic Press (New York), 1-47.

De Boor C., 1981. On a max-norm bound for the least-squares spline approximant. In Approximation and Function Spaces Z. Ciesielski (ed.), North Holland (Amsterdam), 163-175.

Friggens N.C., Emmans G.C., Veerkamp R.F., 1999. On the use of simple ratios between lactation curve coefficients to describbe parity effects on milk production. Livestock Production Science 62, 1-13.

Garcia S.C., Holmes C.W., 2001. Lactation curves of autumn- and spring-calved cows in pasture-based dairy systems. Livestock Production Science, 68 ,189-203.

Olori V.E., Brotherstone S., Hill W.G., McGuirk B.J., 1999. Fit of standard models of the lactation curve to weekly records of milk production of cows in a single herd. Livestock Production Science, 58 ,55-63.

Ordolff D., 2001. Introduction of electronics into milking technology. Computers and Electronics in Agriculture, 30, 125-149.

Pool M.H., Meuwissen T.H.E., 2000. Reduction of the parameters needed for a polynomial random regression test day model. Livestock Production Science 64, 133-145.

Pravdova V., Walczak B., Massart D.L., Kawano S., Toyoda K., Tsennkova R., 2001. Calibration of somatic cell count in milk based on near-infrared spectroscopy. Analytica Chimica Acta 450, 131-141.

Pulina G., Cappio-Borlino A., Macciotta N., Di Mauro C., Nudda A., 2001. Empirical and mechanistic mathematical models of temporal evolution of milk prodution in ruminants. Rivista di Biologia / Biology Forum 94, 331-344.

Rekaya R., Carabano M.J., Toro M.A., 1999. Use of test day yields for the genetic evaluation of production traits in Holstein-Friesian cattle. Livestock Production Science, 57, 203-217.

Rekaya R., Weigel K.A., Gianola D., 2001. Hierarchical nonlinear model for persistency of milk yield in the first three lactations of Holstein. Livestock Production Science, 68, 181-187.

Salehi F., Lacroix R., Wade K.M., 2000. Development of neuro-fuzzyfiers for qualitative analyses of milk yield. Computer and Electronics in Agriculture 28, 171-186.

Snedecor G.W., Coochran W.G., 1989. Statistical Methods. Eight Edition, Iowa State University Press, Ames, Iowa 50010.

Svennersten-Sjaunja K., Sjaunja L.-O., Bertilsson J., Wiktorsson H., 1997. Use of regular milking records versus daily records for nutrition and other kinds of management. Livestock Production Science, 48, 167-174.

The development of integrated management systems for livestock production

A.R. Frost, D.J. Parsons, A.P. Robertson, C.P. Schofield and K.F. Stacey
Silsoe Research Institute, Wrest Park, Silsoe, Bedford, MK45 4HS, UK

Abstract

Silsoe Research Institute has a research programme aimed at developing integrated closed-loop, model-based, control systems for livestock production. Effort so far has concentrated on developing systems which will integrate the management of growth and pollutant emissions for pigs and poultry. This paper includes a description of the development and testing of a model-based growth controller in eight houses on a commercial broiler farm.

Keywords: livestock management, model-based control

Introduction

The objective of a livestock production system is to achieve an acceptable economic performance, without compromising animal welfare or the environment. Performance is controlled by regulating inputs such as nutrition and housing conditions. The problem is that the effects on performance of making changes to any of the inputs can be difficult to predict. For example growth, health, welfare and environmental emissions all depend on the animals' supply of nutrients. It is therefore not possible to manage growth by controlling nutrition without affecting health, welfare and emissions. Traditionally, livestock management has been based on the judgement and experience of the stockman who has to estimate the likely effects of any action. This leads to dilemmas. A change of diet may increase growth rate and enable a delivery date to be met, but will the increased feed cost be justified, and will the change of diet make the animal too fat? Such dilemmas arise because each of the individual processes is controlled separately. The connections between the various aspects of process management need to be strengthened through the development of integrated management systems, which control simultaneously more than one, and ideally all, interrelated processes involved in livestock production.

Control system design

The simplest form of control system (open loop) is represented by the upper level of Figure 1.

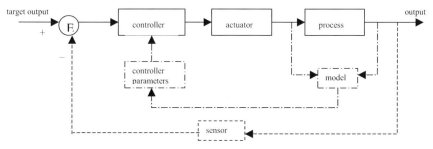

Figure 1. Process controllers: —— open loop control; ------ sensor added to give closed loop control; ·——·— model added to give model-based closed loop control.

The user sets the input to the controller, which then controls the process through the actuator, with no feedback. Most livestock production control systems operate like this. In the case of rearing animals for meat, the input is a desired growth rate; the controller is the farm manager; the actuator is the nutrition supply system; the process is the animal; and the output is the resulting growth rate. However there are many factors (eg disease, or unfavourable environment) which may prevent the animals from achieving their potential, and targets will be missed. This is a general problem with open-loop control systems; the output is free to drift. A typical livestock production enterprise relies on a set of such open-loop control systems, each of which controls only part of the overall process. The enterprise relies for success on the skill of the stockman and the tolerance and resilience of the stock. With the diminishing supply of skilled stockmen exacerbating the difficulties, it is not surprising that many producers fail to meet the increasingly stringent requirements of their customers. The problems inherent in the open loop control system can be reduced by introducing a feedback loop, in which the value of the output is measured, compared to the input, and the difference between them (the error) used to control the actuator. This is illustrated in the second level of Figure 1.

In livestock production, a human manager frequently assumes the role of the controller in determining the required magnitude of the correcting action. In the case of rearing meat animals, feedback control can be effected by weighing the animals at, say, weekly intervals so that deviations from the expected growth curve can be detected and the manager can take some corrective action by varying the nutritional inputs to bring the animals back on course to reach their target weight. Generally this decision will be based on experience and intuition, and consequently levels of success are variable.

The above approach presupposes that the process that is being controlled behaves consistently and repeatably. In practice this assumption is frequently unfounded, especially if the process involves animals. One solution to this problem is to incorporate a model of the process in the controller. The model can then be continuously revised to reflect changes in the real process, and can be used to recalculate suitable controller parameters. This is shown in the final level of Figure 1. The model of the process, which is driven by the process input and output, is used to calculate suitable values for the controller parameters. In this way the characteristics of the controller are responsive to the behaviour of the process; if the process changes, the controller changes accordingly.

In summary, any livestock production system can be represented as a set of complex, variable, interconnected processes each of which is under independent open-loop control. The solution to the problems caused by this type of control is to introduce management systems in which the controllers of the various processes are integrated so that the production system is managed as a whole, with as many of the controllers as possible being closed loop, to counter output drift, and incorporating process models to accommodate process inconsistencies.

An ideal integrated management system for a livestock production enterprise would be one which controls all relevant processes. For example if the purpose of the system were to regulate nutritional input in order to control animal growth and pollutant emissions, the controller would calculate input values which would enable growth and emissions criteria to be satisfied simultaneously. If there were conflict between the different criteria, a hierarchy of criteria would be applied to ensure that the highest priority objectives were achieved. In the growth versus emissions example, the best approach might be to give priority to growth, but to make inputs subject to limits calculated to ensure that given emission levels were not exceeded. Greater integration would be achieved if the system were also to control the environment in the animal house by including variables such as heat input and ventilation rate as inputs to the system and including, in the controller, models of the effects of these variables on growth and emissions.

Since the ultimate objective of the integrated management system is to improve the economic performance of the enterprise, it is desirable to include economic models in the controller to ensure that, for example, optimal growth was not achieved at the expense of profitability. If growth rate or timeliness of delivery could be improved by increasing a component of the food supply, the increased value of the animal would have to be compared with the extra costs incurred to see if there were an overall economic benefit. Taking precedence over all other operations in the controller would be a set of limits on each input to ensure that high standards of stockmanship were maintained and that the animals' welfare was not compromised.

Progress towards the development of integrated management systems for livestock

Silsoe Research Institute has a research programme aimed at developing integrated closed-loop, model-based, control systems for livestock production. Effort so far has concentrated on developing systems which will integrate the management of growth and pollutant emissions for pigs and poultry.

Poultry management system

Progress so far includes developing and demonstrating the performance of a novel growth controller and simultaneously monitoring aerial pollutant emission responses to nutritional inputs (Frost et al, in press). The growth controller required a suitable model which was capable of responding realistically to a wide range of inputs. A semi-mechanistic growth model was developed in which growth is predicted from feed intake and feed composition each day. A model adaptation mechanism was included to accommodate variations between flocks due to factors beyond the scope of the model, such as genetic variation, parent flock age and flock health. It was concluded that the most effective method was to optimise a single parameter added to the model, which could be interpreted as the overall diet digestibility or metabolic efficiency. This was optimised so that the residual mean square error between the actual weights as measured by automatic bird weighers and the growth as predicted by the growth model is minimised for the previous 14 days.

All of the experimental work carried out to develop and test the controller was done on a commercial broiler farm consisting of eight identical, modern houses, each containing approximately 34,000 birds. Each of the houses was fitted with a commercially available broiler nutrition management system (Filmer, 2001). This consisted of a feed system capable of supplying a blend of two feed components with differing compositions. In the original, commercial form of the management system, the manager decided the feed quantity and composition to be supplied on a given day. To inform the manager's decision, the system used a look up table of the daily nutrient requirements of growing broilers, to calculate the blend of the two components that should deliver the required nutrient intake for that day. A series of trials was carried out to compare the performance of this original system to that of the new model-based controller. When using the original system, the manager was at liberty to accept or adjust the calculated diet, whereas the new controller's calculations were implemented without modification. Practicalities dictated however that they could only be updated three times per week, with a 24-hour lag, rather than the ideal of once per day with no lag.

Figure 2 shows some results from one of the trials, which was designed to test the ability of the controller to grow birds to a target weight. For example in House 3 pullets were grown under the control of the manager according to standard practice. In House 5 pullets were grown using the new controller. Neither of the houses achieved its target in this trial, but it can be seen that the performance of the controller was comparable to that of the manager, which was a significant achievement given the experience of the manager and the lack of experience with the new controller.

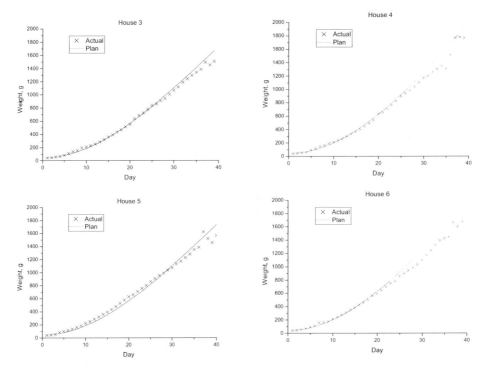

Figure 2. Example results from a trial to illustrate the ability of the new controller to grow birds to a target weight. Houses 3 (pullets) and 4 (cockerels) were grown according to standard practice. Houses 5 (pullets) and 6 (cockerels) were grown by the controller.

It was clear from the trials that automatic growth control based on regulation of diet composition is feasible. The quality of growth control that can be achieved will depend on the extent to which feed intake can be predicted or controlled. Control of intake would be the ideal. However this strategy may not always be acceptable to the grower, who may associate intake control with restriction of intake and growth rate, which they would wish to avoid. Research is required to investigate this supposed association. In the absence of intake control, the next best strategy is to make intake as consistent as possible from one day to the next, because variability in intake makes growth control more difficult.

A fully automatic online version which provides fully automatic, real time control of broiler growth has subsequently been implemented and tested successfully on farms. It allows daily updates with no lag.

Four of the houses used for the growth control experiments were instrumented to monitor the aerial emissions of ammonia, dust and odour (Robertson et al., 2002) as a first step in investigating the effects of diet on emissions at a commercial scale, so that in the longer term, emissions control can be integrated with the growth control. Full analysis of the results is complex and will not be attempted here but the work has demonstrated the ability to quantify many of the factors involved in the production of emissions and has provided indicators of the effects of some of these factors on emission levels. In many cases it was found that general direct causal relationships between diet and emissions were confounded by factors such as the incidence of coccidiosis (which is a commonly occurring disease of the intestinal tract), which tended to reduce ammonia emissions. Relationships were found between diet and emissions of dust and odour. Highest dust and odour emissions occurred with the most extreme diets (lowest protein and highest energy), as a consequence of unusually unsettled bird behaviour. However, it is clear that further experimental work is required to develop causal relationships between diet and emissions. In particular, the role of the litter must be investigated in greater detail. Progress in these areas would lead to the development of an integrated system that controls pollutant emissions as well as bird growth.

Pig production management system

Silsoe Research Institute, with the Universities of Edinburgh and Bristol and commercial partners, is developing a management system comprising sensors, suitable nutrition models and feed control mechanisms, aimed at increasing the efficiency of pig production (Whittemore *et al.*, 2001). As with the poultry management system, the approach involves measuring process outputs including pig growth rate, calculating the difference between actual (measured) and optimal (calculated from a model) growth, and adjusting the feed input to minimise the error.

The system for obtaining pig weight is of interest. Rather than using electro-mechanical devices, which present maintenance problems in the hostile environment of a pig pen, the system uses video cameras to take top view images of a pig, from which its weight can be deduced. Figure 3 shows a representation of the type of image that is obtained. It has been shown (Marchant et al 1999) that the area of the plan view, minus the head, is well correlated with the weight of the animal, as shown in Figure 3.

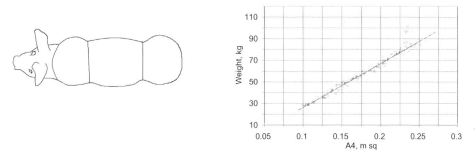

Figure 3. Pig live weight as a function of the plan area A4, which is represented in the plan view of the pig by the area of the three body segments, excluding the head.

It is also possible to make measurements related to the shape of the animal from video images. The possibility that these measurements can provide information relating to the animal's composition is being investigated. If this does prove to be possible it may be that the diet for an individual or groups of pigs could be managed by measuring dimensions relating to their condition, as well as their weight and age. Again, as for the poultry management system the relationship between diet and emissions will be investigated so that the management of emissions can be integrated with that of growth.

Conclusions

Livestock systems comprise sets of complex interconnected processes each with their own outputs eg growth, yield, animal health, welfare and environmental emissions. Livestock management decisions are currently based almost entirely on the judgement and experience of the stockman who has to estimate or guess the likely effects of any control action. Many producers are failing to meet the increasingly stringent requirements of their customers. Other industries faced with similar difficulties have adopted modern methods of process control. Model based control systems are particularly appropriate for accommodating the variability of most livestock production processes. The essential components of a process control system are sensors to measure the relevant variables and models to predict the response of the process to its inputs. An ideal integrated livestock production management system would be one which controlled all relevant processes.

References

Filmer, D. 2001. Nutritional management of meat poultry. In: Integrated Management Systems for Livestock. Edited by C. M. Wathes, A. R. Frost, F. Gordon and J. Wood, Occasional Publication British Society of Animal Science. 2001, No. 28, 133-146.

Frost, A.R., Parsons, D.J., Stacey, K.F., Robertson, A.P., Welch, S.K., Filmer, D., Fothergill, A. Progress Towards the Development of an Integrated Management System for Broiler Chicken Production, Computers and Electronics in Agriculture (in press).

Marchant, J.A., Schofield, C.P., White, R.P. 1999. Pig growth and conformation monitoring using image analysis. Animal Science, 1999, 68, 141-150.

Robertson, A.P., Hoxey, R.P., Demmers, T.G.M., Welch, S.K., Sneath, R.W., Stacey, K.F., Fothergill, A., Filmer, D., Fisher, C. 2002. Commercial-scale studies of the effect of broiler-protein intake on aerial pollutant emissions. Biosystems Engineering, 2002 82 (2) 217-225.

Whittemore, C.T., Green, D.M. and Schofield, C.P. 2001. Nutrition management of growing pigs. In: Integrated Management Systems for Livestock. Edited by C. M. Wathes, A. R. Frost, F. Gordon and J. Wood, Occasional Publication British Society of Animal Science. 2001, No. 28, 89-95.

Acknowledgements

The projects aimed at developing integrated management systems for poultry and for pigs are funded by the UK Department for Environment, Food and Rural Affairs (DEFRA).

Information monitoring system for surveillance of animal welfare during transport

G. Gebresenbet[1], G. Van de Water[2] and R. Geers[2]
[1]*Dept of Agric Eng, Swedish University of Agricultural Sciences, Box 7032, 750 07 Uppsala, Sweden*
[2]*Laboratory for Quality Care in Animal Production, Zootechnical Centre, Katholieke Universiteit Leuven, Bijzondere Weg 12, B-3360 Lovenjoel, Belgium*
Girma.Gebresenbet@lt.slu.se

Abstract

Transport in general compromises animals' health and welfare, meat quality, increases the risk of spread of infectious diseases over large distances, and also degrades the environment in terms of pollution emanating from vehicles.

Currently, no continuous information is available on (a) the climatic conditions, i.e., temperature, relative humidity, and level of gases in the loading compartment, (b) vehicle performance (particularly vibration), (c) driving routes and performances, and (d) animal behaviour when subjected to uncomfortable conditions during transport.

In line with the above objectives, instrumentation of different categories and logistical and control system has been developed and tested has been developed..

With the surveillance system it could be possible to trace all animals from the farm to the abattoir while animal welfare can be monitored by measuring climatic conditions in the vehicle and behavior, which gives an additional guarantee to the consumer.

Key words: Animal welfare, animal transport, monitoring system.

Introduction

The transport of animals is an important component in the production system and welfare of the society as a whole. It is steadily increasing both on national and international levels in relation to marketing systems. Today, both within and between European countries and between European Union and non-EU countries, transport of cattle, pigs, sheep and goats occurs on a large scale. The animals are transported either from farm to slaughterhouse or through a market where they are off-loaded, handled and re-loaded. During road transportation livestock are exposed to a variety of potential stressors such as heat, cold, poor air quality, vibration, motion of the lorry and noise, etc. Many of these factors reduce the welfare and health of the animals and also decrease product quality and may even cause death. Moreover, transport increases the risk of spread of infectious diseases over large distances, and degrades the environment in terms of pollution emanating from vehicles.

Besides the improvement of vehicle design and handling methods, continuous and reliable measurement and reporting of stress inducing factors and stress response parameters, and continuous observation of animals are necessary and essential to improve animal welfare and the quality of meat.

Currently, no on-line information is available on (a) the climatic conditions, i.e., temperature, relative humidity, and level of gases in the loading compartment, (b) vehicle performance (particularly vibration), (c) driving routes and performances, and (d) animal behaviour when subjected to uncomfortable conditions during transport.

New welfare regulations will impose surveillance systems so that information on the quality of transport conditions is available. Moreover a route description is useful not only for optimisation of transport logistics, but also in relation to estimating the risk to food hygiene and food safety, including traceability of individual animals.

The objective of the current work is to develop an information monitoring system for the surveillance of animal welfare during transport. In line with this objective, it was necessary to develop instrumentation of different categories to study air quality, vehicle performance, animal responses in terms of physiological and behavioural alteration during handling and transport from farms to abattoirs, and to transfer information to an on-line control station.

Development of animal data monitoring system

On the basis of the problem described above, a transport surveillance system has been developed (Geers et al, 1997) which integrates the following information (Figure 1): individual identification of animals, unloading place and time, temperature and movement. These data are collected by telemetry and GPS, and are transmitted to a dispatch centre by GSM. Hence, information is available on-line and on disk, so that the driver can be informed and corrected at the spot. This system will be installed on different vehicles for cattle transport, so that the hardware and the collected information can be validated. Further, advice will be generated for vehicle manufacturers, hauliers, farmers, slaughterhouses and retailers.

Huysmans et al. (1999) described the surveillance system and discussed the results of a few trials in practice. The system has two elements: an automated telemetric collection of data in the vehicle and wireless transmission to the data base station. The mobile configuration employs a mobile PC (PC-M), which collects and temporarily stores data that are continuously generated by three inputs: animal identification, animal monitoring (body temperature) and geographical positioning. At regular intervals (e.g. every 5 minutes), the stored data are transmitted using a GSM device (Global System for Mobile communication). Signals received by the base station of the GSM-network are further transmitted through the GSM- and PSTN-networks (Public Switched Telephone Network) to the stationary computer (PC-S) of the data base station. In the present set-up this was the laboratory; in practice this could be the Veterinary Service. Here, all data are stored and processed.

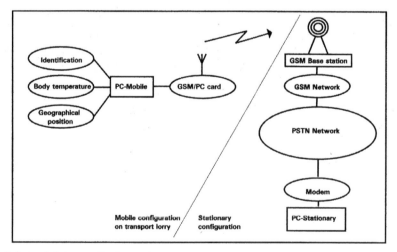

Figure 1. Animal data monitoring system.

For animal identification TIRIS® passive transponders integrated in ear tags were chosen for financial and practical reasons (Geers et al., 1997). The small size and lightweight of a passive transponder were considered to be suitable for this purpose. However, the reading distance of passive transponders appeared too low for continuous data collection from all the animals, particular if the orientation of the transponder to the antenna was less optimal.

Continuous monitoring of body temperature was carried out using the Televilt® RX-900-system (Anonymous, 1996), which employs active transmitters implanted in the neck-region of the animal. Another possibility to connect the transponder with the animal is to enclose the transponder in a bolus and within the animal's stomach (only possible with ruminants). An active transponder needs an internal power source. Although long-life batteries are generally utilised, they require replacement, add weight and are relatively expensive. However, valuable monitoring information in many cases can only be measured on a continuous basis by using a battery.

Geographical positioning of the lorry was determined with a Garmin® GPS 35 device (Anonymous, 1994), placed on the roof of the vehicle. The mobile telephone was a GSM device, which was connected to the PC-M via a modem card. Power supply for all elements of the mobile configuration was either a rechargeable internal battery of the device/system itself or external power supplied by the battery of the vehicle. The PC-S was connected to the PSTN-network with a Belgacom modem.

After starting-up, data are collected and transmitted automatically at pre-defined intervals. Unsuccessful transmission is automatically followed by consecutive attempts with 1 minute intervals until transmission succeeds. Standard compression/decompression procedures for data transmission are included in the software program. For data transmission, a connection between the modems of both PCs has to be established ('hand-shaking'). Received data are stored in ASCII-files and can be processed afterwards using packages such as Excel® and SAS®. Moreover, geographical positions received can be displayed on the PC screen using a digital map (Digimap®).

Ten calf transport studies were followed in September 2002, with the prototype GPS-GSM system in order to test this system under commercial cattle transport conditions. During start up of the system the transmission interval was set at 5 minutes. Before the activation of the GPS-system, general data on the loading procedure were entered into the mobile computer, the loaded animals were scanned by their electronic ID-chip and the geographical locations were determined using GPS signal receiver. All these data were transmitted as a whole to the stationary computer with the GSM-system. At that moment, the base station knows the name and address of the farmer, which animals are loaded and the exact global position of the truck. Then, the GPS-system is activated and the coordinates are transmitted every 5 minutes to the stationary computer where the position of the truck can be followed online throughout the total transport time. A good installation of the antenna is essential for optimal connection with the satellites. Regarding the position of the truck towards the satellite, data can sometimes not be transmitted. After arrival at the slaughterhouse, the GPS-system is inactivated. Again, general data on the unloading procedure is entered into the mobile computer, the unloaded animals are scanned and GPS-coordinates are determined. These data are then transmitted to the stationary computer. All the data from one transport journey can be saved into one file, which can be stored and checked on the stationary computer.

Complementary system

An instrumentation system was developed at the Engineering Department of Swedish University of Agricultural Sciences, SLU, to carry out the measurements of the parameters mentioned earlier and additional parameters simultaneously and continuously during transport from the farms to the abattoir (Gebresenbet and Eriksson, 1998).

The instrumentation may be classified into four groups. Instrumentation for measuring: animal behaviour (digital video), heart rate, transport route, geographical location, vibration sensors mounted both on vehicle and animals, climatic conditions (temperature and humidity), emissions, and information transmission from vehicle to stationary database.

All instrumentation groups were monitored using on-board portable computers from the cabin of the vehicle.

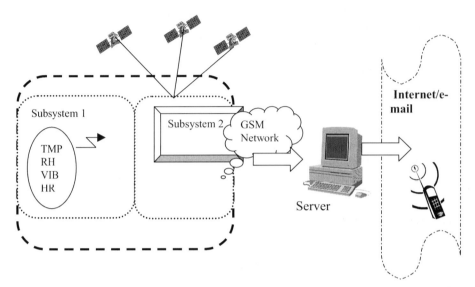

Figure 2. Wireless transport data transmission. TMP, RH, VIB, and HR denote temperature, relative humidity, vibration and heart rate respectively.

The components of the transport surveillance system shown in Figure 2 has two components: (a) Subsystem 1, integrated sensors and data transferring components in the animal loading compartment of the vehicle (information on individual identification of animals, air quality (temperature, relative humidity, emissions), vehicle's and animal vibration and behaviour of the animals, loading and un-loading place and time, and route tracing); (b) Subsystem 2, information storing and data transfer unit in the cabin. Subsystem 2 is also integrated with GPS (to measure geographical location of farms, abattoirs and transport route) and GSM module.

Data transfer from subsystem 1 to subsystem 2 is wireless, and the from subsystem 2 transfer to the server using GSM. Hence, information is available on-line and on disk, so that the driver can be informed and corrected at the spot. It may be noted that sufficient data (that was not transferred to the control centre) are stored in the component to be used if necessary. Another instrumentation package that comprises sensors for heart rate and vibration on the animal has been integrated. These sensors can be mounted on animals and the data is transferred to a database through a wireless network. 19 transports of cattle from farms to abattoirs have been followed and to test the system in Figure 2.

Results and discussions

The results showed that the collection and transmitting of disease and welfare related data (i.e. animal identification, body temperature and geographical position) is technically feasible during transport without major problems and without substantial loss of data. Subsequent storage and processing in the data base station was also possible. Hence, on-line surveillance and monitoring of animal transport and vehicles are possible. At any moment the location and the status of animals and vehicles can be known. Nevertheless, the study indicated also some fields for necessary improvement before the use on large-scale can be considered.

During the 10 transport journeys more than 90% of the data was transmitted correctly. The loss of data was caused by bad contact between the GPS antenna and the satellite when, for example, the truck drove underneath a bridge at the moment of connection and detection. No transmission problems or loss of data have been encountered with the GSM-system. The transmission of body temperature data can still be improved. Transmission difficulties were detected between the Televilt reader and the mobile computer.

Nevertheless, the knowledge and the technique are available and operational to create a commercial model.

Concluding remarks

Using the developed system, accurate measurement can be made and this enables optimization of the handling and transport system to improve animal welfare and environment.

The field measurement and the on-line data transmission system performed satisfactory and hence transport companies, abattoirs and other relevant organizations can use the system. Advice may be generated for vehicle manufacturers, haulers, farmers, slaughterhouses and retailers.

With the surveillance system it could be possible to trace all animals from the farm to the abattoir while animal welfare can be monitored by measuring transport performance and animal conditions gives an additional guarantee to the consumer. This information is also important for the management of the slaughterhouse in order to determine lair age time so that meat quality can be improved.

References

Anonymous (1996) RX-900 receiver and data acquisition system. Televilt International AB, Lindesberg, Sweden, 28 pp.

Anonymous (1994) GPS smart antenna technical specification. Garmin, Lenexa, KA, USA, 20 pp.

Gebresenbet G, and Eriksson B.1998. Effect of transport and handling on animal welfare, meat quality and environment with special emphasis on tied cows. SLU, Dept of Agric Engng, report 233, 1998

Geers R., Puers B., Goedseels V. and Wouters P. 1997. Electronic identification, monitoring and tracking of animals. CAB International, Wallingford (Oxon), UK, 156 pp.

Huysmans K., Saatkamp H.W., Goossens K., Van Camp B., Gorssen J., Rombouts G., Vanthemsche P. and Geers R. 1999. Electronic identification and the use of a surveillance system for animal transports. Proceedings of the 7th Annual Meeting of the Flemish Society for Veterinary Epidemology & Economics. 28/10/1999, Antwerp, Belgium, 42-51

Acknowledgement

The research has been financed by EU within the project: **QLK5-1999-01507, CATRA,** *"Minimising stress inducing factors on cattle during handling and transport to improve animal welfare and meat quality"*

Operation of electronic identification devices in northern winter climate

H.E.S. Haapala

MTT Agrifood Research Finland, Agricultural Engineering Research (Vakola), Vakolantie 55, FIN-03400 Vihti, Finland

hannu.haapala@mtt.fi

Abstract

The aim of the project was to evaluate electronic identification (EI) in a northern winter climate characterized by low temperatures down to -50 °C and rapid and frequent fluctuations (+5 °C to -25 °C). The work was based on the I.D.E.A. project (IDentification Electronique des Animaux: basis for the future implementation of the Electronic Identification System in livestock of the European Union) of EU (Joint Research Centre, Ispra, Italy). I.D.E.A. suggests requirements that might be inadequate in northern climate. The project gave information on the actual operating conditions especially as regards animals kept in uninsulated loose housing. The results enhance JRC's work in defining test procedures and standards. They also give authorities, slaughterhouses and farmers indications of the possible new requirements for production conditions and buildings.

Keywords: electronic identification, cattle, cold climate

Introduction

During the last few years several research projects on livestock electronic identification (FEOGA, AIR2304, I.D.E.A.) have been performed in EU countries. These projects have come to a general conclusion that the electronic identification system is an efficient and reliable method for the traceability of the animals from birth to the slaughterhouse (Rossing 1999, JRC 2002).

The I.D.E.A. project that ended on December 2001 was a large-scale project lasting four years and including approximately one million animals in six EU member states. It was started because of new legislation proposals regarding livestock identification in EU. However, none of the Northern European countries participated in the project, mainly because, at that time, they had only recently joined the EU.

In the Northern European countries livestock are kept under cold conditions, characterized by temperatures down to -50 °C and rapid and frequent temperature fluctuations between +5 and -25 °C. It was anticipated that the results of the ongoing I.D.E.A. project could make proposals that might be inadequate in a northern cold climate (Ribó et al. 2002).

The main objective of this Finnish project was performance evaluation of the electronic identification devices in the above climate. The project was also set up to give information on the actual operating conditions, especially with regard to animals kept in uninsulated loose housing. Finally, the results could enhance JRC's work in defining appropriate test procedures and standards for the RFID devices. (Haapala 2001, Haapala & Havento 2002, Haapala et al. 2002, Ribó et al. 2002)

Materials and methods

EI devices complying with the ISO 11784 (code structure) and 11785 (technical concept) standards were tested in the field on four farms with ca. 270 cattle. Reference tests were done in climatic chambers. Electronic ear tags and ruminal boluses were used as transponders. Both static and dynamic reading methods were tested. To achieve this, hand-held readers and portable stationery readers were tested.

The reference tests were first started in the climatic chambers at the TEMPEST Laboratory of the JRC Ispra, Italy. Selected pieces of equipment were tested mainly according to JRC´s standard test procedures. In addition to standard tests some additional ones were performed according to the Finnish environmental conditions. In reference tests no ruminal boluses were tested, as ambient conditions do not affect their performance. The tested equipment in Ispra were:

- Allflex standard electronic eartag (JRC IDEA certificate No. 11/1997)
- Allflex portable reader (JRC IDEA certificate No. 050/1997)
- Gesimpex Hokofarm Portoreader portable reader (JRC IDEA certificate No. 08/1997)
- Datamars Isomax III portable reader (JRC IDEA certificate No. 035/1997)
- Gesimpex F100 stationary reader (JRC IDEA certificate No. 12/1997)
- Gesimpex F200 stationary reader (JRC IDEA certificate No. 46/1998)
- Gesimpex GO3C stationary antenna (JRC IDEA certificate No. 13/1997)

In addition to above mentioned equipment the following boluses were used in field tests in Finland:
- Alfa Laval Aleis ceramic bolus (JRC IDEA certificate No. 066/1998)
- Allflex Innoceramics ceramic bolus (JRC IDEA certificate No. 074/1999)
- Gesimpex Rumitag bolus (JRC IDEA certificate No. 037/1997)

Eartag operation

First eartag operation in -40 °C was tested. In a climatic chamber selected eartags (10 Allflex standard electronic eartags, JRC IDEA Certificate no 011) were tested at - 40 °C for 96 hours (according to IEC 68.2.1 standard). During the test, each eartag was read inside the climatic chamber using a Datamars Isomax III portable reader.

Portable readers

The number of readings and the "reading autonomy" of portable readers at -25 ° C were defined. Reading autonomy was considered as the time after introducing the reader inside the chamber until it was impossible to read the bolus code. Three portable readers were introduced from ambient temperature inside a climatic chamber at -25 ° C with their batteries fully charged. At that temperature, a Rumitag bolus was continuously read.

For the third reference test the selected portable readers were placed, batteries fully charged, at - 10 °C for 96 hours (according to IEC 68.2.1 standard). During the test the readers were checked every day by reading the ID code of a Rumitag bolus

In order to study the recovery time from -25 °C to ambient temperature (i.e. the ability of the portable readers when transferred from -25 °C to ambient temperature to read again a transponder), the following special test was conducted: the readers were placed for 48 hours at -25 °C then quickly placed at room temperature. Pressing continuously their reading switch, it was recorded after how much time they were able to read again a Rumitag bolus and to display clearly the ID number.

Stationary readers

The two stationary readers with their antennae were placed at -40 °C for 96 hours (according to IEC 68.2.1 standard). The temperature decreasing speed (from ambient to -40 °C) and increasing time (from -40 °C to ambient) was set to 2 hours. During the test, the readers were continuously powered and a Rumitag bolus was read twice a day.

One of the important aspects to be considered on the readers' performance is the temperature variation with a short time period. Due to the important temperature variations occurring in Finland, the following test was conducted on the two stationary readers: two readers (with their antennae) were submitted during 10 days to a thermal cycle (Figure 1). During the test, the readers were continuously powered and a Rumitag bolus was read regularly.

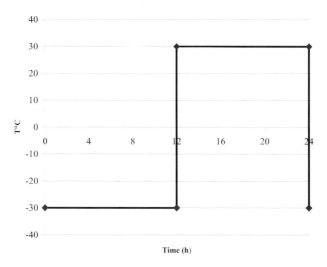

Figure 1. Thermal cycle -30 °C/+30 °C for stationary readers.

Field tests

In field tests in Finland, all animals on the selected four farms were equipped with transponders. A total of 273 beef and dairy cattle were electronically identified with ruminal boluses (n=165) and electronic eartags (n=108). Animals were located in four farms with different breeding and temperature conditions. (Table 1)

Table 1. Number of animals identified on each farm and temperature conditions. Very Cold Conditions: outside without any insulation (VCC), Cold Conditions: inside without heating system (CC) and Warm Conditions: inside with heating system (WC).

Farm	Breeding	Tag	Temperature conditions			Total
			VCC	CC	WC	
Suckler cow unit, Tohmajärvi Experimental Farm	Beef cattle	Eartags	36	65	7	108
		Bolus	5	8		13
Sampo Rauma	Beef calves	Bolus		56		
Kitee Learning Centre		Bolus			14	
Suitia Research Farm		Bolus			42	
Total			41	169	63	273

The researchers visited the farms regularly and read the tags with handheld and portable readers. The information was stored in a database, which followed the approved data dictionary standard. The success in identifications was recorded together with the environmental conditions (temperature and relative humidity). Environmental measurements were done with recording instruments to chart the temperature history of the devices.

Necessary data were communicated to JRC. The animals to be slaughtered during the project period were followed and identified in the slaughterhouse as far as it was technically possible. The used ear tags and boluses were collected for later inspection.

Results

Eartags

The first reference test (-40 °C for 96 hours) with the selected eartags was successful: no mechanical or electronic problems occurred.

Portable readers

Reading autonomy of portable readers at -25 °C was quite good, except for Gesimpex Hokofarm Portoreader which operated satisfactory for only 11 minutes. The difference between readers in the number of successful readings was also quite high (Table 2).

The reading efficiency of portable readers at -10°C was acceptable, except for Datamars Isomax III in which the display was all the time unreadable even at this moderate temperature (Table 3). After being for 48 hours at -25 °C the portable readers recovered in 9 to 24 minutes so that they could read a Rumitag bolus and show the ID clearly on their displays (Table 4).

Stationary readers

Both tested stationary readers, Gesimpex F 100 and Gesimpex F 200, performed perfectly when tested in -40 °C for 96 hours.

The two stationary readers submitted to a 10-day thermal cycle were operational. The Rumitag bolus could be read throughout the test time.

Field tests

In field test all the transponders worked satisfactory. The readers, on the other hand, were quite different from each other. (Table 5)

Table 2. Reading autonomy of portable readers at -25 °C.

Reader	Number of readings	Autonomy (min)
Allflex Portable Reader (JRC Cert. 050)	790	25[1]
Datamars Isomax III (JRC Cert. 035)	230	20[2]
Gesimpex Hokofarm Portoreader (JRC Cert. 008)	112	11[3]

[1]Frost on the display.
[2]After 6 minutes, display response slow and not as clear as at ambient temperature.
[3]After 8 minutes, display response slow and not as clear as at ambient temperature.

Table 3. Reading efficiency of portable readers at -10°C.

Date	Hour	Allflex	Isomax III	Hokofarm
11-29-99	13:00	1	2	1
11-29-99	14:55	1	2	1
11-30-99	08:10	OK	3	OK
11-30-99	09:45	OK	2	OK
11-30-99	11:15	OK	2	OK
11-30-99	13:20	OK	2	OK
11-30-99	15:50	OK	2	OK
12-01-99	07:50	OK	2	OK
12-01-99	12:00	OK	2	OK
12-01-99	14:15	OK	2	OK
12-01-99	15:50	OK	2	OK
12-02-99	07:30	OK	2	OK
12-02-99	10:39	OK	2	OK
12-02-99	13:45	OK	2	OK
12-02-99	15:55	OK	2	OK
12-03-99	07:45	OK	2	OK
12-03-99	09:39	OK	2	OK
12-03-99	12:05	OK	2	OK

1: Limited readability of the display.
2: Quite impossible to read the bolus ID number on the reader's display.
3: Battery charger connected to the reader.

Table 4. Recovery time of readers from -25 °C to ambient temperature.

Reader	Recovery time (min)	Ambient temperature (°C)
Allflex	9	24.9
Isomax III	24	20.6
Hokofarm	11	25.3

Differences in reading time and physical dimensions and field shape of the antenna caused great variation in reading work. When using handheld readers with short antennas and short reading distance the work postures were quite difficult. The work was also potentially dangerous, especially in slippery surfaces that are common in cold environment. The casing material of some readers was not suitable for cold environment since it turned slippery in low temperatures. There were also no carrying straps in the readers to hold them firmly during reading so that they could easily be dropped. It was also observed that in almost every reader there were too low-level audible and/or visible signals indicating a successful reading.

In stationary readers there were some annoying faults in the antennas. The antennas were very sensitive to electromagnetic disturbances and required precise installation to avoid malfunction. There was also a lot of trouble with the connection software to external computers.

Table 5. Summary of the readings with the reading date, reading type, the reading efficiency and T/RH conditions.

| Farm | Reading type / date | | | | |
	1 day	1 month	7 months	Every 7 months	Every 7 months
Tohmajärvi Exp. Farm	21-12-99 Dynamic 100% (48/48) -16 °C, 75%	22-3-00 Dynamic 100% (95/95) +3 °C, 70%	13-7-00 Dynamic (n=101) Static (n=7) 100% (108/108) +23 °C, 80%	12-12-00 Dynamic 100% (101/101) +8 °C, 98%	29.3.2001[1] Dynamic 100% (99/99) -1 °C, 83%
Kitee Learning Centre	21.12.1999 Static 100% (14/14) -6 °C	22.03.2000 Static 100% (10/10) +4 °C	All animals slaughtered		
Sampo Rauma	22-3-00 Dynamic 91% (41/45) +4 °C	13-7-00 Dynamic 100% (19/19) +23 °C	7-3-01 Static 100% (2/2) -6 °C	All animals slaughtered	
Suitia Research Farm	30-3-00 Static 100% (82/82) Dynamic 0 % +13 °C, 57%	18-5-00 Static 100% (82/82) Dynamic 0 % +18 °C, 53%	19.12.00 Dynamic (n=17) Static (n=65) 100% (82/82) +13 °C, 80%	8.3.2001 Dynamic (n=57) Static (n=4) 100% (61/61) +13 °C, 75%	25-4-01 Dynamic 93.4% (57/61)[2]

[1]An additional reading was performed with 100% or reading efficiency (101/101).
[2]Not checked with Portable Reader.

In slaughterhouses it was quite easy to retrieve the boluses and ear tags. Data handling and integration to existing registers was quite easy.

Discussion and conclusions

Most of the problems encountered were due to other reasons than the cold environment. It can be concluded that the operation and functioning of the electronic identification devices used in this study were satisfactory. If some precautions are met the devices can be used even for cattle kept at extreme temperature and humidity conditions. No problems were encountered with the eartags or boluses. The portable readers, however, showed some problems in cold conditions, especially with displays and battery operation. Static readers were operational.

Usability of the portable devices in cold conditions needs further research. The poor ergonomics of handling, short battery life in autonomous mode and display problems need to be solved before the full implementation of the electronic identification system in northern countries starts.

It would be rational to use the same tag for all the appliances where animal identification is needed so that e.g. the automatic feeding systems would use the system as well. This would also reduce the possibilities of electromagnetic disturbances between the two systems

The EI system, if implemented, has wide effects on the whole production system in EU. There is great variation in local circumstances. Thus, before implementation, the readiness of the whole production chain needs to be analysed in order to minimize disorder. Management issues such as arrangements in animal traffic seem to be the most tedious challenges to meet. Farms tend to lack good solutions for catching the animals for tagging so new solutions have to be developed and tested in practical environment.

Acknowledgements

This project was funded by Joint Research Centre of European Union and Finnish Ministry of Agriculture and Forestry.

References

Haapala, H. 2001. Eläinten elektroninen tunnistus - apuväline tulevaisuuteen. (Electronic identification of animals - a tool for future). Lihatalous 6.

Haapala, H. & Havento, J. 2002. Electronic identification of cattle in Finland. In: Proceedings of the 3rd Scientific and Practical Conference. June 5-6 2002. Russian Academy of Agricultural Sciences. Saint-Petersburg. Vol 2.

Haapala, H., Havento, J., Kangasniemi, R. & Peltonen, M. 2002. Eläinten elektroninen merkintä elintarvikeketjussa. (Electronic identification of animals in food chain). Maataloustieteen päivät 2002. Finnish society of agricultural sciences. Electronic publication: http://www.maataloustieteellinenseura.fi/mtp2002

Ribó, O., Havento, J., Haapala, H., Kangasniemi, R., Mainetti, S. & Korn, C. 2002. Electronic Identification of Cattle in Finland: Operation and Functioning of Electronic Identification Devices in Northern Cold Climate. Technical Note. Draft version 2. European Commission. Institute for the Protection and the Security of the Citizen (IPSC) Non-Proliferation and Nuclear Safeguards Unit.

JRC 2002. Monitoring of Livestock (IDEA). CODE ISIS-11. Electronic publication: http://www.jrc.cec.eu.int/download/workprogram2001-en.pdf. p. 141.

Rossing, W. (ed.) 1999. Electronic animal identification. Computers and electronics in agriculture. 24, 1-117.

Evaluation of a dry matter intake model for individual cows

I. Halachmi[1], Y. Edan[2], U. Moallem[1] and E. Maltz[1]

[1]*Agricultural Research Organization, the Volcani Center, P. O. Box 6, Bet Dagan 50250, Israel*
[2]*Department of Industrial Engineering and Management, Ben-Gurion University of the Negev, Be'er Sheva 84105, Israel*
halachmi@volcani.agri.gov.il

Abstract

A model predicting the individual dry matter intake (DMI) of dairy cows was evaluated. The input parameters are body weight and milk yield, which are both measurable on-line in an commercial dairy farm. The model output is voluntary DMI (kg per day) for each individual cow, which can be used in nutritional calculation for the individuals. The new model was statistically validated by comparison with the NRC model. In one herd, 76% cows passed the statistical test, compared with 33% when the NRC model was used; in a second herd, 11 cows (50%) passed the test with the new model, and only 1 with the NRC model.
Evaluation with a larger number of cows is necessary to determine the usefulness of the model in programming individual feeding of high-yield cows.

Key words: dairy cow; dry matter; feed intake; feed ration; milking robot

Introduction

The voluntary feed intake of individual dairy cows is an important variable in dairy management, and it becomes crucial to the maintenance of optimal nutrition when concentrates are allocated individually through the computer-controlled self-feeders that are an essential part of robot-milking systems (Halachmi et al., 2002). Individual dry matter intake (DMI) measurements can be done for cows in tied-stall barns or in small-scale operations (Halachmi et al., 1998), but most cows are fed TMR from mixer wagons, so that individual intakes cannot be determined directly, and modeling is the only practicable way to address the problem (National Research Council (NRC), 2001, pp 3-12). There are several approaches to modelling DMI (Mertens, 1987; Roseler et al., 1997a, b) and it is generally accepted that short-term (daily) individual DMI evaluation necessitates a sacrifice of model accuracy. Nevertheless, preliminary attempts suggested that modelling individual DMI on a daily, or even real-time basis is feasible (Halachmi et al., 1997). The original version of the new model has been tested on a new data set, and it has been updated by the inclusion of the effect of milk fat content and the addition of a new smoothing algorithm. The purpose of the present study was to evaluate the model in calculating the DMI from the absolute values of daily milk yield (MY) and cow body weight (BW), as well as from the relative values of their daily fluctuations.

Materials and methods

Animals. Two herds, with total of 60 cows were used in the experiments at the Bet Dagan experimental farm. In the first experiment, in 1997 39 high-yielding multiparous Israeli-Holstein cows, which had calved between November 1996 and February 1997, were housed in loose covered pens with adjacent yards. A second almost identical experiment was carried out during 2001, this time with 21 cows. The cows were offered a TMR containing corn grain, barley grain, sorghum grain, wheat silage, corn silage, and wheat bran; the nutrient contents were NE_L 1.67 Mcal/kg, CP 16.9, ADF 18.8, NDF 34.2, P 0.5 and Ca 0.8 % of DM. These are the constituents of a common

Israeli diet, described by Moallem et al. (2000). All feeds were mixed and fed once daily from a mixing wagon. The duration and feed intake of every visit were recorded by a 'real-time control system for individual dairy cow food intake' as described previously (Halachmi et al., 1998). The daily intake of each cow was recorded during 1 year following parturition. The cows were weighed with an automatic electronic scale three times daily, after every milking, and their milk yields were recorded electronically.

Daily milk yield, BW and DMI of the individual cow are noisy and variable (Maltz and Metz, 1994; Halachmi et al., 1997; Maltz et al., 1997), so that it is difficult to discern a trend. To overcome this problem we implemented an old smoothing algorithm (Whittaker, 1923) in Matlab (Eilers, 1997), with third-order differences and λ = 10000. Figure 1 shows the fluctuating raw data for an individual cow, with fitted trend lines.

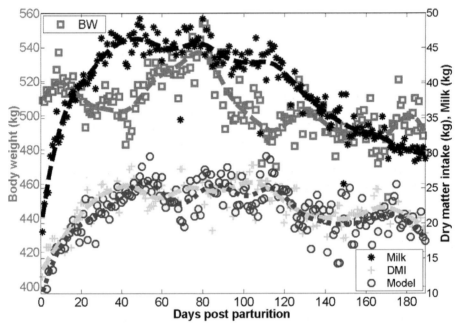

Figure 1. Daily feed intake (kg DMI/day, +), milk yield (kg/day, *) and body weight (kg, □) for an individual cow. Model (o) and smoothing trend lines (----) are also shown.

Regression coefficients. We found it more useful to use the relative values of the independent variables than their absolute values

$$DMI = \left[\frac{MY_0}{BW_0} \quad \frac{MY_{-1}}{BW_{-1}} \quad \frac{MY_{-2}}{BW_{-2}} \quad BW_0 \quad difBW \quad fat \right] b + e \qquad (1)$$

Where the column vectors are:
1 DMI, the predicted voluntary dry matter intake for the individual cow;
2 MY_0/BW_0, the current day's (day 0) milk yield (kg) divided by the cow's body weight (kg) measured at the same time;
3 MY_{-1}/BW_{-1}, the previous day's (day -1) milk yield (kg) divided by the cow's body weight (kg);

4 MY_{-2}/BW_{-2}, the milk yield that was measured two days previously (day -2), divided by the cow's body weight;

5 BW_0, the current body weight (day 0);

6 $diffBW = BW_{-1}/BW_0$, the body weight change since day -1;

7 fat, the percentage of milk fat as measured in the last milk recording.

The small ratios MY_i/BW_i (8) are multiplied by 100 and BW_0 is divided by 100. The regression coefficients, b, were calculated for each day. In the first herd, the 19 cows with the longest lactation periods were used for calculating the coefficients; there was a separate set of six regression coefficients for each day; e is the residual error. The correlation coefficients of the DMI, averaged over all the days, were 0.44, 0.43, 0.42, -0.36, 0.04, and -0.01, for the chosen regression parameters:

$$\frac{MY_0}{BW_0} , \frac{MY_{-1}}{BW_{-1}} , \frac{MY_{-2}}{BW_{-2}} , BW_0 , difBW , fat \qquad (9)$$

respectively.

Model validation. Let X_i and Y_i denote the actual and model outputs, respectively, in day i. In *regression analysis* the ideal model would mean $X_i = Y_i$, $\forall\ i$. This equality implies that the regression line $Y = \beta_0 + \beta_1 X$ should have $(H_0:)\ \beta_0 = 0\ and\ \beta_1 = 1$, i.e., a unity-gradient (45°) line passing through the origin (zero intercept). For the theory behind the associated *F-test* we refer to Kleijnen and van Groenendaal (1992),i pp. 209-210, for the equations we refer to Kleijnen et al.,1998 equation 4 and 5. The computer code implementation is given below:

```
B=regress(Y,[ones(size(X)) X]);        % returns the vector of regression coefficients,
ForcY=[ones(size(X)) X]*B;             % Forecasting
SSEfull=sum((Y-ForcY).^2);             % Kleijnen et al. EQ 4
SSEreduced=sum((Y-X).^2);              % Kleijnen et al. EQ 5
n=length(X);                           % F-statistic with two degrees of freedom
Fstatistic=((n-2)/2)*(SSEreduced-SSEfull)/SSEfull;  % Kleijnen et al. EQ 5
```

Results

The model predicted the voluntary DMI, in kilograms per day, for each cow in the herds. It can be seen (Table 1) that the F-statistic and the mean error (ME) were generally lower in calculations with the new model than in those with the NRC model. The mean absolute error (MAE) was higher with the new model because of the wide fluctuations of the MAE in the course of the lactation period. The results from the 2nd herd were identical (Table 2). The results of the statistical F-test suggest that, under the limited number of cows tested in this trial, the new model gave better predictions than the NRC model, and this interpretation was supported by the visual analysis in Figure 1, in which the model trend line covers that of the actual data through almost the whole lactation period and in Figure 2.

Discussion

Like the NRC model this model uses performance data (BW, MY, and milk fat), avoiding nutritional and nutrition related variables. However, this model includes also the ratio of MY to BW which is an efficiency-related variable, as well as "historic" (previous two days) values of the above. This is very important, because at least part of the daily voluntary DMI fluctuations are the result of compensation for "historic" intake. After all, our diurnal definition is not exactly the cows' choice. Eating a big meal before midnight or delaying it to after midnight, because of some routine delay, can make a significant difference in "daily" DMI measured at midnight. The performance of this model is encouraging enough to stimulate further research to reach a sufficient data base to challenge in time the NRC (2001) model.

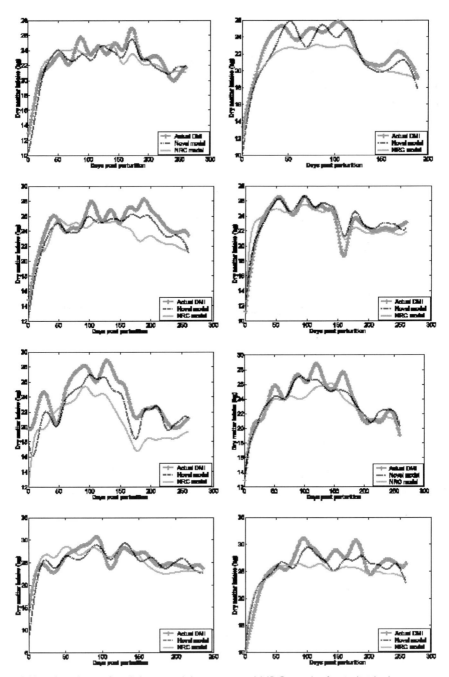

Figure 2. Visual analysis of real data, model outputs and NRC results for individual cows.

Data from 17,087 cows were used for evaluation and development of the NRC (2001) equations. Thus, further research is needed, to provide more data for evaluating the new model before it can be operated routinely on commercial farms, embedded in the self-feeder or robot software

Perhaps the use of regression coefficients that vary during the course of the lactation gives the model its strength. A cow changes physiologically from the early to the later stages of lactation, and the NRC model handles this phenomenon by applying a nonlinear function, e^{aT+b} that smoothes the entire curve. The new model may be dynamically applicable to the daily feed allocation to each individual cow because: (1) it incorporates daily changes in milk production and body weight; and (2) it changes the coefficients the course of the lactation.

The fact that the data in the present study were collected from cows that were undergoing several nutritional and hormonal treatments (Moallem et al., 2000), and the model preformed well suggests that the chosen parameters and methodology are on the right tract.

Table 1. Statistical tests; comparing the new model with the NRC model. Both models predict dry matter intake of each individual cow kept in herd number 1.

Cow	F-test		ME		MAE	
	New	NRC	New	NRC	New	NRC
1580	34	14	-0.74	-1.24	3.33	2.62
1608	54	251	-1.83	-1.25	3.11	2.4
1622	94	368	-2.29	-1.61	3.06	2.4
1644	51	81	0.33	0.21	3.08	1.88
1665	236	773	4.77	4.12	5.26	4.48
1667	137	525	-3.51	-2.36	3.94	2.57
1707	74	451	0.35	0.12	2.96	2.27
1718	239	673	-3.3	-3.16	4.87	3.63
1733	47	344	1.5	1.83	4.21	3.59
1749	70	120	0.79	0.83	2.71	2.23
1759	123	434	2.54	3.17	3.66	3.5
1760	170	330	2.92	3.02	4.41	3.94
1761	375	1545	7.25	6.46	7.69	6.93
1773	258	729	6.28	6.75	6.93	6.96
1775	24	101	0.3	0.57	2.62	1.89
1814	42	136	-0.69	-0.28	2.46	1.76
1821	42	83	0.31	0.15	2.59	2.33
1825	134	243	1.73	1.62	3.74	2.6
1833	15	206	0.72	1.53	2.33	2.04
1846	13	43	-0.75	-0.09	2.95	1.6
average	112	373	0.83	1.02	3.80	3.08
sum	2232	7450	16.68	20.39	75.91	61.62
pass the test[1]	16 (76%)	7(33%)				

[1]Number of cows that pass the statistical test (F<199). $F_n;2;0.995 \approx 199$ (99.5% significant level, n days in lactation, two degrees of freedom).

Conclusions

The model predicted the voluntary feed intake of individual cows. After validation with a larger number of cows, the model could be useful when individual feeding is needed for high-yield cows, under circumstances resembling those of this trial. The new model might be used either on a stand-alone basis or incorporated into a milking robot software, to facilitate the improvement of individual feeding management based on a concentrate self-feeder.

Table 2. Statistical tests; comparing the new model with the NRC model. Both models predict dry matter intake of each individual cow kept in herd number 2.

Cow	F-test		ME		MAE	
	New	NRC	New	NRC	New	NRC
1906	393	2958	-0.54	0.07	5.49	4.73
2003	427	2131	4.05	3.77	5.04	4.73
2124	67	427	0.75	1.44	2.5	2.26
2148	233	539	-0.45	0.91	2.51	2.27
1942	159	795	-2.69	-1.46	3.84	2.52
2048	437	3257	-0.77	-0.15	5.64	4.87
2136	38	189	-0.42	-0.48	2.21	1.44
2153	475	1442	3.75	4.25	4.66	4.84
1852	257	866	0.73	2.58	2.54	2.93
1955	250	470	-2.91	-2.46	3.65	3.45
2063	88	349	-2.04	-1.05	3.48	2.16
2141	467	1098	1.8	2.26	2.62	2.62
2160	97	297	-2.05	-0.63	3.47	1.6
1871	99	244	1.07	1.56	2.47	2.29
1962	105	474	0.25	1.04	1.94	2.15
2072	94	312	-0.43	-0.96	3.54	3.43
2145	101	563	0.93	2.18	3.15	2.69
1892	119	249	-2.14	-1.57	3.64	2.32
2002	230	397	-0.13	-0.18	3.19	2.24
2118	77	327	1.36	0.66	2.6	2.01
2147	245	933	2.22	2.69	3.15	2.95
average	212	872	0.11	0.69	3.40	2.88
sum	4458	18317	2.34	14.47	71.33	60.5
pass the test	11 (50%)	1				

References

Eilers, P.H.C. 1997. Smoothing with Matlab. Pages 1-8 in Proc. Benelux Matlab Users' Conf., October, Amsterdam, the Netherlands.

Halachmi, I., E. Maltz, J.H.M. Metz, and S. Devir. 1997. The body weight of the dairy cow: II. Modeling individual voluntary food intake based on body weight and milk production. Livestock Prod. Sci. 48:244-246.

Halachmi, I., Y. Edan, E. Maltz, U.M. Peiper, I. Brukental, and U. Moalem. 1998 A real-time control system for individual dairy cow food intake. Comp. Electron. Agric. 20:131-144.

Halachmi, I., J.H.M. Metz, A. van't Land, S. Halachmi, and J.P.C. Kleijnen. 2002. Optimal facility allocation in a robotic milking barn. Trans. ASAE 45: 1539-1546

Kleijnen, J.P.C., and W.J.H. van Groenendaal, Simulation: a Statistical Perspective, Wiley, Chichester, UK, 1992.

Kleijnen, J.P.C., B.Bettonvil, W.J.H.van Groenendaal, Validation of Trace-Driven Simulation Models: A Novel Regression Test, Managment Science. Vol 44, No. 6, June 1998

Maltz, E., S. Devir, J.H.M. Metz, and H. Hogeveen. 1997. The body weight of the dairy cow: I. Introductory study into body weight changes in dairy cows as a management aid. Livestock Prod. Sci. 48:175-186.

Mertens, D.R. 1987. Predicting intake and digestibility using mathematical models of ruminal function. J. Anim. Sci. 64:1548-1558.

Moallem, U., Y. Folman, and D. Sklan. 2000. Effects of somatotropin and dietary calcium of fatty acids in early lactation on milk production, dry matter intake, and energy balance of high-yielding dairy cows. J. Dairy Sci. 83:2085-2094.

National Research Council (NRC). 2001. Nutrient Requirements of Dairy Cattle. 7th rev. ed. National Academy Press. Washington, DC, USA

Roseler, D.K., D.G. Fox, L.E. Chase, A.N. Pell, and W.C. Stone. 1997a. Development and evaluation of equations for prediction of feed intake for lactating Holstein cows. J. Dairy Sci. 80:878-893.

Roseler, D.K., D.G. Fox, A.N. Pell, and L.E. Chase, 1997b. Evaluation of alternative equations for prediction of intake for Holstein dairy cows. J. Dairy Sci. 80:864-877.

Whittaker, E.T. 1923. On a new method of graduation. Proc. Edinburgh Math. Soc. 41:63-75.

Improvement of teat cup attachment in automatic milking systems by using teat coordinates

J. Harms and G. Wendl
Bavarian State Research Center for Agriculture, Institute of Agricultural Engineering, Farm Buildings and Environmental Technology, 85354 Freising, Germany
jan.harms@lfl.bayern.de

Abstract

In automatic milking systems a quick and sure attachment of the teat cups is important for system capacity. An investigation was undertaken, to determine if it is possible to decide whether a found teat position is plausible, before the teat cup is attached. It was based on 55,225 milkings of 94 different Simmental cows which were milked by an automatic milking system. Using the animal and the lactation number as parameters, 90.9% to 92.4% of variation in the vertical teat positions could be explained, depending which teat was concerned. With the target of reaching a high specificity of 99.99%, 37% to 47% of all "wrong attachments" were predicted correctly only by reference to the teat coordinates before attaching the cup.

Keywords: automatic milking, teat coordinates, teat cup attachment, udder height

Introduction

With automatic milking systems quick and sure attachment of the teat cups is important because the time for teat cup attachment and the number of failed attachments are factors among others that influence the system capacity (De Koning et al, 2000; Sonck & Donkers, 1995). Attaching teat cups has greatly improved in recent years, but in some cases the attachment still fails. Normally, the average teat positions of a number of successful milkings are used for roughly locating the teats. Then an optical or ultrasonic system searches for the exact teat position and the teat cup is attached (Artmann, 1997; Wendl & Schön, 2002). After that the system has to wait for a feedback like milk flow or constant vacuum to decide whether the attachment was successful or not. This "waiting time" can take more time than the attachment itself.

Because there is only little literature available on how teat coordinates change during lactation, from cow to cow or with different milking intervals (Miller et.al. 1995, Geidel & Graff 2002) this investigation was undertaken to analyse the teat coordinates in a robotic milking system.

In a second step these results were analysed to determine if it is possible to decide whether a found teat position is plausible, before the teat cup is attached and so save the "waiting time".

Materials and methods

The investigation was based on 55,225 milkings or 220,900 cup attachments of 94 different Simmental cows on a research farm between August 2000 and August 2002. The lactation number of the cows varied from one to seven. During the investigated period on average 47.4 cows were milked per day with a frequency of 2.7 milkings per cow. Only cows with data for more than 100 consecutive days were taken into account.

They were milked by an automatic milking system, type "Fullwood-Merlin" installed in May 1998, which is comparable in many parts to the "Lely-Astronaut" system especially concerning the robot arm. The teats are located by a pivoting laser unit on the robot arm. If the bottom of the teat is found, the cup is attached.

For every milking the system records the coordinates and the milking time of each teat. The vertical teat coordinates (distance of the bottom of a teat to the floor = teat height) of all successful attachments (milk yield > 0 kg) were compared to those where the robot attached the cup but no milk flow occurred. In the following these cases are called "wrong attachment". In total 1,520 "wrong attachments" were observed which were 0.7% of all investigated attachments. This happened at 1136 milkings which were 2.1% of all investigated milkings.

In a first step the influence of the single animal, the lactation number, the day in lactation and the milking interval on teat height were analysed. For statistical analysis of covariance the general linear model procedure (GLM) of SAS (SAS 8.01) was used. Four models were tested:

$$y_i = \mu + \alpha_i + e_i \tag{1}$$
$$y_{ij} = \mu + \alpha_i + \beta n_j + e_{ij} \tag{2}$$
$$y_{ij} = \mu + \alpha_i + \beta n_j + \gamma x_j + e_{ij} \tag{3}$$
$$y_{ij} = \mu + \alpha_i + \beta n_j + \gamma x_j + \delta z_j + e_{ij} \tag{4}$$

with: y_{ij}: Height of the teat
μ: Intercept
α_i: Influence of the cow
βn_j: Regression of y on lactation number (n)
γx_j: Regression of y on day in lactation (x)
δz_j: Regression of y on milking interval (z)
e_j; e_{ij}: Error

In a second step the difference between the actual height of each teat and the average of the last ten successful milkings was analysed for all attachments in order to find a rule to detect incorrect teat localisations. To evaluate whether it is possible to predict the success of teat cup attachment before attaching the cup, different limits for this difference were tested.

Results

Variation of vertical teat position

Only small variation coefficients were found in the vertical teat positions of all successful milkings. Averaging the mean values of teat height and the variation coefficients for each animal shows that teat height varies only in a small range (Table 1). The position of the front teats is about 7 - 8 mm higher than the position of the rear teats.

Table 1. Vertical teat positions and variation coefficients of all successful milkings (mean values of the individual animal were averaged).

Teat	vertical teat position [mm]	variation coefficient [%]
Right front	415.5	5.3
Right rear	407.5	5.8
Left front	416.0	5.3
Left rear	409.1	5.8

Analysing the height of a single teat with the general linear model (GLM), the animal and the lactation number had the most influence (Table 2). Using these parameters, the model explained 90.9% to 92.4% of variation, depending which teat was concerned. Taking the day of lactation and the milking interval into the model, R^2 increased only very little.

Table 2. R^2 of different tested models to explain vertical teat positions.

Teat	R^2 model 1 with -cow	R^2 model 2 with -cow, -number of lactation	R^2 model 3 with -cow -number of lactation, -day of lactation	R^2 model 4 with -cow, -number of lactation, -day of lactation, -milking interval
Right front	0.792	0.909	0.910	0.910
Right rear	0.797	0.923	0.923	0.924
Left front	0.791	0.910	0.911	0.911
Left rear	0.796	0.924	0.924	0.925

Optimising teat cup attachment

Based on the finding that vertical teat positions of successful milkings show only small changes during lactation and from milking to milking, it was examined if this fact offers the possibility to predict "wrong attachments" before attaching the cup. Therefore the differences in teat height of the actual milking to the last 10 successful milkings were analysed.

More than 95% of all successful attachments had differences of less than 20 mm. Regarding the attachments with no milk flow the differences were much higher. Only 17% to 24% of them had a difference of less than 20 mm, depending which teat was concerned (Figure 1).

To determine if it is possible to predict "wrong attachments" before attaching the cup different limits for the difference of the actual teat height to the last 10 successful milkings were tested. The aim was to reach a high specificity (at least 99.99%). At the same time the sensitivity (cases of predicted "wrong attachments" compared to actual "wrong attachments") should be as high as possible. The specificity of 99.99% was reached when using the rule: "If the difference to the last ten successful milkings is bigger than 60 mm then the actual attaching procedure is assumed to be unsuccessful". Using this limit 37% to 47% of all "wrong attachments" were detected before attaching the cup (sensitivity) depending which teat was concerned. Sensitivity and specificity varied depending of the chosen limit as can be seen in Table 3. With a lower limit the sensitivity improved, but the specificity was decreasing.

For illustration: Within the investigated 55,225 milkings or 220,900 attachments a limit of 60 mm led to 26 attachments which would have been restarted because of a supposed wrong teat position even though the position was correct. These 26 wrong decisions did influence 18 milkings ("Milkings with a needless restart"). On the other hand 667 of 1520 "wrong attachments" were detected correctly. In these cases the waiting time for feedback of the system could be saved because the localisation of the teat would restart immediately.

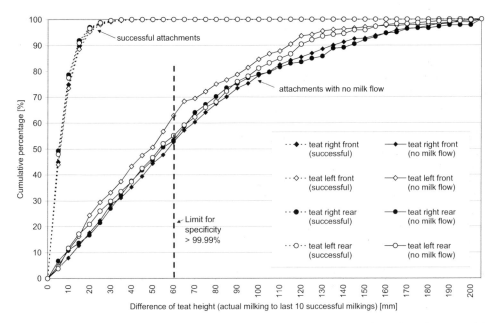

Figure 1. Differences of teat height (actual milking to last 10 successful milkings) successful attachments and attachments with no milk flow.

Table 3. Sensitivity, specificity and milkings with a needless restart at different limits for the difference in teat height (n = 55,225 milkings).

Limit [mm]	Sensitivity [%]				Specificity [%]				Milkings with a needless restart
	right front	right rear	left front	left rear	right front	right rear	left front	left rear	
40	64.73	62.40	56.76	62.67	99.87	99.93	99.83	99.94	184
45	60.58	58.22	52.52	57.53	99.94	99.96	99.94	99.97	80
50	55.60	54.32	49.34	53.42	99.97	99.98	99.97	99.98	40
55	52.28	49.30	43.24	47.95	99.98	99.98	99.98	99.98	28
60	47.30	46.80	37.14	44.86	99.99	99.99	99.99	99.99	18
65	42.74	41.23	31.56	40.75	99.99	99.99	99.99	99.99	8
70	39.63	35.93	30.50	37.67	100.00	99.99	100.00	100.00	4
75	35.89	32.87	27.85	33.90	100.00	99.99	100.00	100.00	4
80	32.57	29.81	24.93	31.85	100.00	100.00	100.00	100.00	4

Conclusions

In the investigated herd teat height changed only very little during lactation and from milking to milking. Using a linear model only based on cow and number of lactation to explain the vertical position of each teat, R^2 of more than 90% were found. Other factors like day of lactation or milking interval had only a small influence on teat height within the investigated 94 cows.

Based on this, a plausibility check for the teat position before attaching the teat cup is possible. A specificity of 99.99% combined with a sensitivity of 37% to 47% was reached depending which teat was concerned.

This offers the possibility to restart searching the teat when a wrong position is indicated, while taking only a low risk of making a wrong decision (only in 26 of 220,900 attachments a needless restart was recommended by the system). This can save the time that is normally needed to wait for a feedback from the system like milk flow or constant vacuum. It can be a further small step towards an improvement in speed and reliability, combined with low cost.

In this investigation only the vertical teat coordinates were used to detect a supposed wrong teat localisation and no difference was made between deviations upward or downward. The prediction might be improved by calculating an individual range for a "normal" teat position for each cow starting with default values at the begin of lactation. Another possibility might be the additional use of the horizontal positions of the teats and the distances between them.

In this investigation teat cup attachment with no milk flow was observed only in 2.0% of all milkings and in 0.7% of all attachments. So the possible effects on system capacity were only small. In other herds with more problems with attachment there might be larger effects. Especially if there are some cows with long hairs at the udder, straw at the udder or other problems the system capacity can benefit from an improved attachment. The costs for this technical improvement are very low, because all sensors that are necessary for a decision are already implemented in the system.

References

Artmann, R. 1997. Sensor systems for milking robots. -In: Special Issue: Robotic milking, edited by Ordolff, D. Computers and Electronics in Agriculture, Volume 17. pp. 19-40

De Koning, K., Ouweltjes, W. 2000. Maximising the milking capacity of an automatic milking system. -In: Proceedings of the international symposium for robotic milking, edited by H. Hogeveen and A. Meijering, Lelystad 2000. pp. 38-46.

Geidel, St., Graff, K. 2002. Morphologische Merkmale des Euters, insbesondere der Zitzen bei Milchrindern (Morphological characteristics of the udder, especially of the teats, of dairy cattle). -In: Rekasan-Journal 9 (2002) Heft 17/18. pp. 63-66.

Miller, R.H., Fulton, L.A., Erez, B., Williams, W.F. and Pearson, R.E. 1995. Variation in distances among teats of Holstein cows: Implications for automated milking. -In: Journal of Dairy Science 78: 1456-1462.

Sonck, B.R., Donkers, J.H.W. 1995. The milking capacity of a milking robot. -In: Journal of Agricultural Engineering Research 62. pp. 25-38.

Wendl, G., Schön, H. 2002. Technik in der Rinderhaltung (Techniques for cattle husbandry). -In: Jahrbuch Landtechnik (Yearbook Agricultural Engineering) 14, edited by J. Matthies, Münster 2002. pp. 175-181.

Individual identification of dairy cows by their voice

Yoshio Ikeda[1], Gerhard Jahns[2], Takahisa Nishizu[1], Kunio Sato[3] and Yoshinari Morio[3]
[1]Kyoto University, Graduate School of Agric., Dept. of Environmental Science and Tech., 6068502 Kyoto, Japan
[2]Federal Agricultural Research Center(FAL), 38116 Braunschweig, Germany
[3]Mie University, Faculty of Bio-Resource, 5148507 Mie, Japan

Abstract

The objective of this study was to determine the extent to which a cow can be recognized by spectral analysis of her voice independently of her distance from the sound receiver and their relative attitudes.
This was achieved through analysis of the short-time variance of the cow's voice, to generate a power/frequency spectrum. As with other biological systems it was found that the power/frequency spectrum could be fitted to a straight line on a log-log chart, which was not affected by the cow's spatial relationship to the sound receiver.
However, simultaneous monitoring of the voices of three cows showed that the system could not separate their voice spectra unambiguously. Other means must be explored for cow identification.

Keywords: cow's voice, linear prediction model, recognition, mathematical ethology

Introduction

Animals have a central nervous system and exhibit autonomous behaviour in response to their environmental conditions and their physical states, such as sickness, oestrus or hunger (Xin et al, 1989, Jahns et al, 1997, Bradbury and Vehrencamp, 1998, Hopp et al, 1998). Therefore, it is academically attractive research to understand animal behaviour through the computer. From the practical point of view, and of course, for automation of animal husbandry for precision livestock farming, it is necessary to understand animal behaviour and condition by some means, to realize the precision breeding of the individual animal. The behaviour of the animals can be generally understood through the auditory and visual senses from the viewpoint of non-contact and non-invasive detection. The mathematical ethology for the farm animal may involve these motivations and concepts, therefore we hope that the present research topics should be the sprout of engineering and mathematical animal ethology for the precision livestock industry.
This research was undertaken to establish how far a cow could be identified by voice recognition. If this could be achieved it would have the advantage that the data acquisition system is comparatively simple and low-cost. The problem is that cows moving freely in the yard or pen will not be at a fixed attitude to the sound received. It is therefore necessary to normalize the signal amplitude by some means. The object of this research was to find a method which would compensate for these variations.

Theoretical background

In the analysis of human speech, it is general to assume that the speech signal is modeled by the linear prediction filter and the speech production process can be described by the following (Morishita and Kobatake, 1982, Rabinar and Juang, 1993, Deller et al, 1993).

$$s(n) = \sum_{i=1}^{p} a_i s(n-i) + \Theta' e(n) \tag{1}$$

where $s(n)$ is the digitized voice signal at the sampling time, n, $a_i, i=1, \ldots, p$ is a prediction coefficient, Θ' is a gain of the voice signal producing system including the vocal code to the receiver, and $e(n)$ is the driving signal of the system. By this assumption, the voice characteristics can be described by the coefficients a_i numerically. When the voice producing organ does not change its characteristics during vocalization, the system gain can absorb the variation of the voice loudness due to the change of the relative distance or attitude between the sound source and the receiver. Therefore, we can compare the voice characteristics directly by using the prediction coefficients.

The power spectrum of the voice signal can be given by (Hino, 1986)

$$P(f) = \frac{\Delta t P_m}{\left|1 + \sum_{i=1}^{P} a_i e^{j2\pi f k\Delta t}\right|}$$ (2)

where Δt is the sampling interval of signal and P_m is the expected value of the prediction error.

Experimental conditions

Cattle used for Experiments Three dairy cows were used in the experimental farm of FAL in Germany. The experiments were made for three days in the morning before feeding.

Data Acquisition The vocalization of cow was collected by a condenser microphone with a frequency range between 20 Hz and 20 kHz, sampled at the rate of 48 kHz, converted to the digital signal of 16 bits full scale, and stored in the hard disc of the computer.

Data Processing Since the voice signal of cattle is brief and non-stationary, we have no formal procedure for data processing. In other words, the ordinary digital signal processing technique cannot be applied directly to the voice signal of cattle. In the present paper, we propose a new technique for processing. Figure 1 shows a flow chart of the data processing as explained in the following.

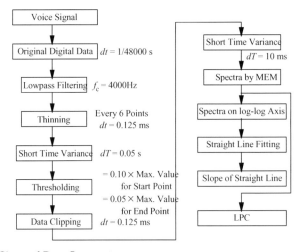

Figure 1. Flow Chart of Data Processing.

Precision lifestock farming

In Figure 2, the total power or variance of each voice signal is shown. The value of the vertical axis has no physical unit, but represents the value proportional to the variance of voice signal during vocalization. The height of each column corresponds to the total power of each voice. The five voice signals with the highest total power (indicated with the downward arrows) were selected for each cow to further discussion.

Because of the too high sampling rate of 48 kHz for the cow vocalization(Ikeda & Ishii, 2001) and the microphone's frequency characteristic, the frequency components higher than 4 kHz were filtered out by the simple digital low-pass filter, and re-sampled at every six points. Hence the sampling rate was reduced to 8 kHz.

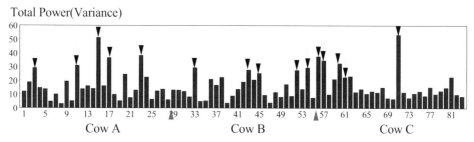

Figure 2. Total power of each vocalization.

In order to realize the exact analysis of voice signal, it is important to detect the beginning of vocalization precisely and objectively (Rabinar& Juang, 1993). From the overall vocalization signal determined manually on the monitor screen and from the audio speaker for re-production of the recorded voice signal in the disc, the real part of vocalization was extracted by thresholding the sequence of variance for the short time of 50 ms as shown in Figure 3. In this figure, the value of variance is normalized by the maximum values of variance of each voice, and C56, for example,

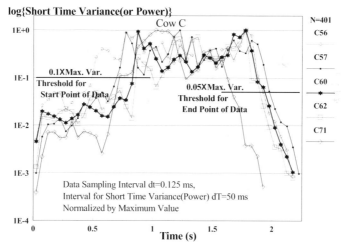

Figure 3. Temporal change of short time variance and thresholding for detection of start and end of data.

in the right column means the 56-th voice of cow C. The threshold for detecting the start of the vocalization is 0.1 and the threshold for the end is 0.05.

The data points corresponding to the interval determined by this thresholding were used for the subsequent computation. This sequence can be considered as the fluctuation of the loudness through vocalization. It and its mirror image about the time axis may constitute the approximation of the amplitude envelope (that is, rough pattern of voice signal). The pattern of the short time variance may reflect the feature of the vocalization of the individual cow as shown in Figure 4.

The spectra of the sequence of short time variance for 10 ms were determined by the Maximum Entropy Method (MEM) for estimating the parameters (Linear Prediction Coding, LPC) contained in the linear prediction filter expressed by Equation (1). The determination of the number of the terms involved in the linear prediction model is of importance, but is very difficult. In this research, the number of terms was determined in the same way as for the MEM spectra to trace the FFT spectra as faithfully as possible, and the number of terms in this research was 7(=MMAX).

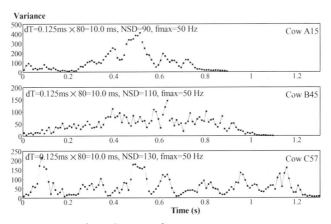

Figure 4. Short time variance of vocalization of cows.

Results and discussion

The spectrum of the short time variance on log-log scale could be fitted to the straight line expressed by $\log P(f) = a + b \log f$ between 1 and 40 Hz as shown in Figure 5. The power spectra of the short time variance may obey the $1/f$ spectral trend on log-log scale like other biological signal. That is, the variation of loudness of vocalization may assume to show the trend in which the power of the spectrum is inversely proportional to the frequency f according to a $1/f^b$ power law (Measurement Encyclopedia). The value of the slope b may be expected to characterize the voice for recognition of individual cow. The example of the fitting results is shown in Table 1 for the 15-th voice of the cow A, 33-rd of the cow B and the 71-st of the cow C. Under this assumption, we try to recognize individual cow with the slope of the straight line fitted to the spectra on log-log scale. Figure 6 shows the result of recognition by the slopes of the log-log spectra. Cows A and B could be recognized, but Cows A and C as well as Cows B and C could not be recognized rightly. In Figure 7, the recognition result is shown, constructing the two-dimensional feature space, which had intended to increase recognition accuracy, with the filter parameter and the slope of the spectra of the short time variance. The filter parameter used in this feature space is the first coefficient of the linear prediction model expressed by Equation (1). Even on the two-dimensional feature space, Cows A and B can be identified, but other combination could not be recognized.

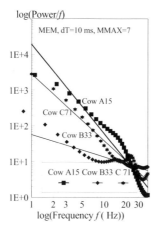

Figure 5. Straight line fitting of spectra of short time variance on log-log scale.

Table 1. Results of straight line fitting.

Cow	Voice	b	r^2
A	15	-2.4958	0.9360
B	33	-0.6277	0.8297
C	71	-1.8597	0.9578

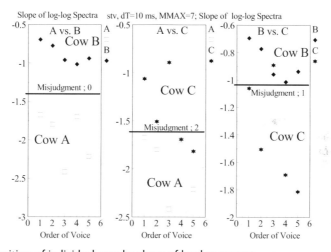

Figure 6. Recognition of individual cow by slope of log-log spectra.

Conclusions

This trial showed that the method cannot be relied upon for clear distinction between cows. Other feature parameters such as the fundamental frequency of the voice signal, could be considered.

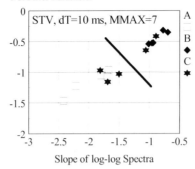

1-st Filter Parameter

Figure 7. Recognition of cows on feature space of filter coefficient and slope of short time variance.

However, when cows perceive the sound of the feeding device at feeding time, they make vocalization at the same time. Therefore it would be necessary to develop data processing techniques to separate the overlapped signal. Since a cow seldom vocalizes in isolation under ordinary conditions, this severely limits the area of application of the method. It is clearly not suitable for traceability purpose, nor for daily monitoring for individual breeding, except in extraordinary physical or psychological conditions. To understand these conditions of the animals through their vocalization, agricultural engineering scientists must collaborate with animal scientists.

The future of identification must lie with facial or other aspects of the cow, for example, a black-and-white pattern that is immutable over its lifetime.

References

Bradbury, L. and Vehrencamp, S.L. 1998. Principles of Animal Communication, Sinauer Associates, Inc.

Deller, J.R., Proakis, J.G. and Hansen, J.H.L.1993. Discrete-Time Processing of Speech Signals. Macmillan.

Hino, M. 1986. Spectral Analysis(in Japanese), Asakura Shoten.

Hopp, S.L., Owren,M.J. and Evans,C.S.(Eds.) 1998. Animal Acoustic Communication, Springer.

Ikeda, Y. and Ishii, Y. 2001. Characteristics of Cow's Voices in Time and Frequency Domains for Recognition. Int. J. of Agricultural ad Biosystems Engineering, Vol. 2, No. 1, 15-23.

Jahns, G., Kowalczyk, W. and Walter, K. 1997. An Application of Sound Processing Techniques for Determining Conditions of Cow, Proc. 4th Int. Workshop on Systems, Signals and Image Processing.

Measurement Encyclopedia, National Instruments http://zone.ni.com/devzone/nidzgloss.nsf/glossary/

Morishita, I. and Kobatake, H. 1982. Signal Processing (in Japanese), SICE.

Rabinar, L. and Juang, B.H. 1993. Fundamentals of Speech Recognition, Prentice Hall.

Xin, H, DeShazer, J.A. and Leger, D,W. 1989. Pig Vocalization under Selected Husbandry Practices, Trans. ASAE, Vol.32, No.6, 2181-2184.

Acknowledgements

This research was supported by the fund for collaboration with Germany of JSPS and Zusammenarbeit mit Japan of DFG. The authors would like to thank for the support given by the governments of Japan and Germany. And also we wish to thank the staff of FAL who gave great support for the experiments in the Institute for Animal Science and Animal Behaviour (Mariensee) of FAL.

Infrared positioning system to identify the location of animals

R. Kaufmann, H. Bollhalder and M. Gysi
Swiss Federal Research Station for Agricultural Economics and Engineering, CH-8356 Taenikon, Switzerland
Robert.kaufmann@fat.admin.ch

Abstract

Animal behaviour is an important criterion when assessing housing systems. Until now behavioural research has been based primarily on direct or video observations. The drawbacks of both methods are high labour input and problems with nocturnal observation.
An electronic monitoring system has been developed, based on video cameras with infrared filters, animal collars for the transmission of infrared impulses and image analysis software. Tests confirmed its accuracy in detection (< 2% errors) and its flexibility in use. One important advantage of this system is that the technical installation has absolutely no influence on the behaviour of the animal.

Keywords: location identification, infrared positioning system, electronic animal monitoring, animal behaviour

Introduction

Animal behaviour is one of the most important criteria when assessing the animal friendliness of a housing system. A factor of interest is the frequency with which the animal group stays in different housing zones. Until now behavioural research has been based primarily on direct observations or video observations. The drawbacks of both methods are high labour input and problems with nocturnal observation. Direct observation can influence the natural behaviour of the animals, particularly when a minimum amount of light is required in nocturnal situations. There is an increasing demand for automatic monitoring systems to carry out rational and cost effective research in the field of animal behaviour.

The Swiss Federal Research Station for Agricultural Economics and Engineering, Tänikon (FAT) has already developed an electronic positioning system (Bollhalder & Krötzl Messerli, 1997). It is based on transmitters worn around the cows' necks, combined with an aerial system embedded in the floor. This was successful in automatically recording the location of a cow in a defined housing area. However, the considerable disadvantages of this positioning system are the major structural expenditure involved in embedding the aerial and the fact that it is restricted to one installation site and cannot therefore be moved to other locations.

In 2001, Haidn monitored the test area with video cameras and determined the location of pigs using image processing techniques. However, it was not possible to relate behaviour to individual animals. The operation of this technique was also relatively unreliable.

The objective of a new development at the FAT was to create a system which could be used for the observation of animals both indoors and out, and which yielded reliable time and space-related information on individual animals.

System Description

The newly developed **FAT - For Animal Tracing 2002**© positioning system comprises the following elements:
• Video cameras fitted with infrared filters (Figure 1).

- Animal collars for the transmission of infrared pulses (Figure 2).
- Image analysis and evaluation software.

A camera mounted 4 metres above the test area covers a range of approx. 8 x 6 metres. In the present layout, a computer station can process the signals from four cameras. This is the equivalent of a test area of around 200 m², or the area occupied by 20-30 cows in a loose dairy housing system. Specially equipped collars emit infrared impulses from individual animals. The transmitter used for animal identification and herd management is mounted on normal cow collars. The signals received by the cameras are evaluated by analysis software according to time and location. The individual sections of floor space to be separately recorded and analysed in a particular experiment can be configured on the PC in any graphic form desired.

With the aid of cameras, the system is able to record the position of up to 100 different animals and to relate the signal to a maximum of four groups. The position of the camera can be adapted according to the question posed. It can be mounted above any area in the housing system. The observation area can be divided into altogether 100 subfields. The lower time resolution is a one minute positioning interval and the spatial resolution is ten centimetres.

The image analysis software is based on applications used in industrial optical process monitoring.

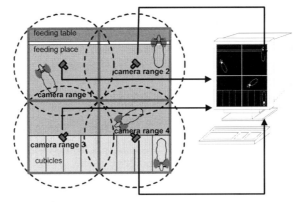

Figure 1. Positioning system diagram.

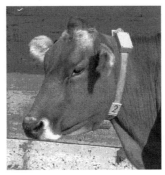

Figure 2. Animal collar transmitter.

Materials and methods

The system is currently in the test phase for checking functional reliability and user friendliness. Weaknesses in the prototype software had to be eliminated. Moreover, it was necessary to remove the initial interference caused by the incidence of sunlight using optimised infrared filters and software measures in the image processing. However, the first results collected during low autumnal light conditions must still be validated during more intensive exposure to the sun (summer).

To determine positioning reliability, data from the FAT 2002 electronic positioning system, differentiated according to exercise, lying and feeding areas, was compared with results from direct observation.

Results

Operation is user-friendly. The desired investigation areas can be adapted to new investigative requirements with a click of the mouse. The whole investigation area is clearly visible on the screen without infrared filters in front (Figure 3).

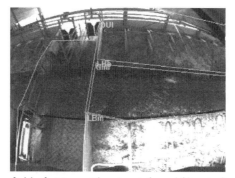

Figure 3. View of a camera field of vision without an infrared filter in front. Two rows of cubicles and the exit area can be seen. The lines denote the defined investigation areas.

During the locating operation, the cattle identified appear on the screen as numbers with times and an indication of position (standing/lying) (Figure 4).

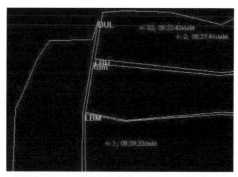

Figure 4. The same image detail with an infrared filter. The cattle located are shown as a number with the time, two in the upper lying area, one in the lower lying area.

Data processing is reliable. Certain evaluation routines are required for user-friendly data handling in Excel. These routines are carried out e.g. by means of macros and have to be adapted according to the question examined.

The system was designed with a target of 98 % system reliability. This means that a maximum of 2 out of 100 animals observed are not identified by the system and can therefore not be recorded and related to a specific area. The reference tests show that this target can be met (Table. 1).

A lower hit rate was observed at the feeding area adjacent to the open external wall. There may be two reasons for this:

1. When the cow is lying, signal transmission may occasionally be interrupted due to the angle of the camera.
2. In the lateral stalls, intensive incidence of sunlight may have caused additional interference.

The absence of wrong animal positioning confirms that the system works reliably.

Table 1. Reliability test of the FAT 2002 electronic positioning system (area with 18 cubicles, herd size of 17 animals, 3 observation series of 3 hours each).

Areas observed	Total number of cow positions observed per area	Of which correctly positioned	Of which wrongly positioned	Of which not positioned	Hit rate
Cubicles at external wall	111	61	0	50	55%
Cubicles in the middle of the stable	158	156	0	0	100%
Passages (lying area)	2	2	0	0	100%
Feeding passage and feeding barrier	446	199	0	247	45%
Lateral passages (drinking facility)	12	12	0	0	100%

As expected, the system had no influence on the behaviour of the observed animals as the wearing comfort of the transmitter collar does not differ from that of the normal transponder collar. The slightly higher weight does not seem to provoke any unusual irritation.

Discussion and conclusions

The **FAT - For Animal Tracing** 2002© positioning system can automatically record and evaluate the locations of individual animals in space and time with high accuracy. This permits the rational observation of behaviour in housing systems.

Initial experience in the field has been positive and has proved that the system functions. Equipped with the appropriate analysis software, control functions can be transmitted to the system as well as recording the desired behavioural parameters. For example, correct herd allocation in the housing area can be monitored with electronic access gates.

The experience gained show that the system offers the following strengths:

• The animal is not influenced by the observation procedure.
• Nocturnal observation is possible without artificial light.

- Animal numbers, groups, and the shape and size of observation areas can be flexibly defined and adjusted to suit the experiment.
- Flexibility of research location. The system supports on-farm research.

The system is being further developed in the following directions:
1. Mobile version: designed to support on-farm research projects. Based on the experience gained in the experimental area of the FAT housing system, there is no doubt that the entire equipment can also be used in comparable situations in practice. It is essential that the ceiling height is sufficient for the installation of the camera.
2. Recording movement in the third dimension: this will make it possible to distinguish between a standing animal and a resting one. This option is already prepared in the transmitter part and on the analysis software side. This will therefore be one of the coming stages of development.
3. Outdoor version: can conceivably be used outdoors if suitably suspended, protected from the weather, and the recording technology adapted appropriately. The appropriate measures have already been taken to reduce the failure rate caused by the influence of sunlight in the stall. There is still some uncertainty concerning positioning reliability when the transmitter is entirely exposed to sunlight. The system could possibly function outdoors, but the relevant trials have yet to be carried out.

References

Bollhalder H., Krötzl Messerli H. 1997. Ein Tierortungssystem zur automatischen Erfassung des Aufenthaltsortes und der Aktivität von Kühen im Laufhof und im Laufstall *[An animal positioning system for automatically recording the location and activity of cattle in the exercise yard and in loose housing]*, Agrartechnische Forschung 3: 2-10.
Haidn B., Freiberger M. 2001. Automatic image analysis of animal behaviour taking rearing piglets as an example. Construction, Engineering and Environment in Livestock Farming, Hohenheim, March 2001: 296-300.

Satellite based spatial information on pastures improves

Australian sheep production

R. Kelly[1], A. Edirisinghe[1], G. Donald[1], C. Oldham[2] and D. Henry[1]
[1]CSIRO Livestock Industries, Private Bag 5, Wembley, WA 6913, Australia
[2]Department of Agriculture WA, Locked Bag 4, Bentley Delivery Centre WA 6983, Australia
rob.kelly@csiro.au

Abstract

Studies have shown that in many years in the winter rainfall regions of southern Australia the amount of pasture grown that is consumed by sheep varies between 20 and 30%, and that increased utilisation could double farm profit. This paper reports how the provision of regular information on pastures over the Internet, generated using satellite imagery, is being used in southern Australia to improve grazing of extensive pastures by sheep.

In 2002, pasture growth rates estimated using satellite sensing explained 66% of the variation in on-ground values. Estimated pasture biomass explained 97% of the variance in on-ground measurements. Access to remotely sensed pasture information was provided via the Internet during the 2002 pasture production season. About two thirds of the users of the websites were farmers. Case studies of four farmers show that they were able to achieve increases in wool production per sheep valued at an extra Au$2.63 to $16.30, plus benefits in decreased labour requirements and greater confidence to exploit the technology on a whole farm basis.

Keywords: satellite, pastures, sheep, cattle

Introduction

The capacity of Australia's agricultural industries to continue to remain viable and improve is increasingly affected by the farmer's ability to make timely decisions. Improved utilisation of pastures by the 50 million sheep and cattle across southern Australia provides such an opportunity, as it is generally very low. Michael et al. (1997) estimated that in many years the amount of pasture that is consumed by sheep is between 20 and 30% of what is grown. Economic analyses estimate that better utilisation of pastures could double farm profit - for every 10% increase in utilisation, profit could increase by $20/hectare.year.

There has been considerable investment by many Australian organisations into providing the farmer with skills to improve pasture utilisation. Over the past decade we estimate that more than 10,000 farmers have attended courses, but a recent survey found that only 45% of attendees were using the skills gained to manage their pastures to improve animal performance. Sneddon et al. (2000) conclude that the slow adoption of pasture management techniques may be attributed to lack of farmer confidence in quantifying feed available, and lack of time available to assess pastures across the whole farm. Our experience with farmers suggests fortnightly pasture biomass assessments alone across a 1500 ha property would take ~2 days, and still only provide a retrospective measure of pasture growth rate. The paper reports on the provision of information over the Internet on pasture biomass (www.pgr.csiro.au; www.spatial.agric.wa.gov.au/foo) generated from NOAA AVHRR, Landsat TM and SPOT satellite imagery, including its accuracy and how it is being used to improve sheep and wool production in southern Australian. Pasture growth rates were also offered in 2002 through a commercial e-commerce portal - The Farmshed (www.thefarmshed.com.au).

Materials and methods

The technology to estimate pasture biomass and growth rate has been developed and calibrated since 1995 in the south west of Western Australia (Edirisinghe *et al.* 2000; Edirisinghe *et al.* 2002), which has a typical Mediterranean climate of a wet winter and spring, and dry summer, with pastures based on annual plant species. Monthly estimates of paddock biomass (kg green dry matter/ha) and weekly estimates of pasture growth rate were used to investigate their potential to help manipulate and improve wool and meat production on farming properties (Henry *et al.* 2002; Oldham *et al.* 2002; C.M. Oldham and S.G. Gherardi *pers. comm.*). Additionally, in 2001 and 2002 the pasture growth rate information was delivered to other Mediterranean regions of Australia (South Australia, Victoria, Tasmania and southern New South Wales). Three facets of this work are reported:

1. the accuracy of the satellite based technology in 2002
2. user profiles for 2002
3. experiences of several landholders in the use of the pasture information

The accuracy of remote sensed estimates of pasture biomass was determined by comparison of average values estimated from satellite observations with those derived from on-ground calibrated visual measurements by trained technicians over parallel transects 30 metres apart and 500 metres long, established in paddocks on four commercial farms in south western Australia. The technicians made observations within 5 days of the date of the satellite pass. Each field transect was sampled 6 times during the 6 month growing season. The method of calibration of visual observations of pasture biomass was derived from that published by Haydock and Shaw (1975) as described in detail in Cayley and Bird (1996).

In the case of measuring pasture growth rates, field observations were made on 21 farms at monthly intervals using 900 metre transects with 1 m^2 exclosure cages at 100 metre intervals. The observed pasture growth rate for a paddock was calculated as the average difference in pasture biomass within 10 pasture cages divided by the number of days between observations (Cayley and Bird 1996). The pasture biomass in each cage was the average of four calibrated visual observations, one in each corner of the cage. The correction to the visual observations of biomass was based on the regression between the technicians' visual observation and the measured oven dried biomass from 10 x 0.1 m^2 quadrats (R^2 for the calibration sets was consistently > 0.85).

Results and discussion

Accuracy of the technology

For pasture growth rates, 66% of the variation in the on-ground observed values were explained by those estimated from the combination of satellite and climate data (Figure 1). Interpolation from the NOAA AVHRR 1 km^2 pixel size of the satellite Normalised Difference Vegetation Index (NDVI) images to farm paddocks, combined with the remoteness of the meteorological stations to the paddocks being studied, are likely factors contributing to this relationship between the on ground observations and estimated pasture growth rates. In 2001, over six farms, we were able to explain 60% of the variance in on-ground observations by estimated pasture growth rate. This compares with an average of 70% in previous years (Edirisinghe *et al.* 2002). We believe that with the advent of new remote sensed data (e.g. from the MODIS sensors on the TERRA and AQUA satellites) substantial improvements in the precision of the estimation of pasture growth rate can be achieved, as the satellites have greater resolution, more frequent overpasses, and more spectral bands to derive information than NOAA AVHRR.

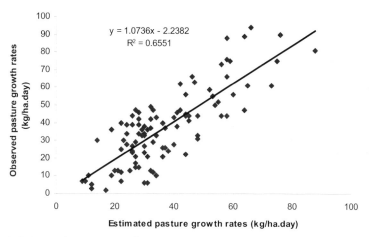

Figure 1. Relationship between Observed and Estimated pasture growth rates in 2002 on 21 farms in south western Australia over the growing season - whole paddock values.

Ninety seven percent of the variation in the observed biomass was predicted, covering a range of 500 to 3500 kg dry matter per hectare, as shown in Figure 2.

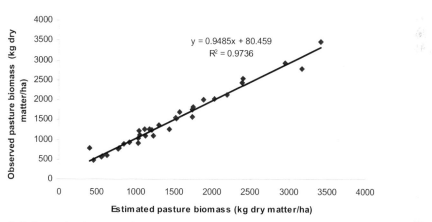

Figure 2. Relationship between Observed and Estimated pasture biomass in 2002 over four farms in south western Australia - transect values.

User profile for 2002

Two pasture information distribution channels to users were piloted in 2002 - the Commonwealth Scientific and Industrial Research Organisation (CSIRO) website (www.pgr.csiro.au), and the commercial website of The Farmshed (www.thefarmshed.com.au). Farmers wishing to access pasture biomass did so via the Agriculture Western Australia's site (www.spatial.agric.wa.gov.au). The login information provided by users of the pasture growth rate sites show a similar distribution in their classification, with about two-thirds being the main target market for this information viz. farmers (Table 1). The CSIRO website had more users from Government Agency's (e.g. Western

Australian Department of Agriculture), undoubtedly reflecting the involvement of these agency's in the on-farm application of the technology (Oldham *et al.* 2002).

Table 1. Profile of users of the Pasture Growth Rate websites - percentage in each classification.

Classification	CSIRO website (n* = 571)	The Farmshed website (n = 2639)
Farmer	65	71
Government Agency	20	6
Educator/student	4	4
Rural Service Provider	3	7
Other	7	12

* number of individual login identities

User experiences

Three farmers (House *et al.* 2002) reported the successful use of pasture biomass and growth rate information to manage wool quality in fine wool sheep flocks. Their approach was based on the work of Thompson *et al.* (1997) who showed that there was a strong positive relationship between pasture biomass and the fibre diameter of wool grown by Merino sheep in spring. The objective of these primary producers was to reduce mean fibre diameter, and increase staple strength in fleeces of young Merino sheep. Overall fleece value per head increased by Au$16.30, Au$8.93 and Au$2.63. Additional benefits from running more sheep on a smaller area of land, so releasing extra hectares for other farming activities, were not measured.

In 2001 in a separate case study (Coole, R. *pers. comm.*), the value of the information on pasture biomass and growth rate was estimated at Au$6-10 per sheep. The ability to capture this benefit was dependent on the satellite technology, because of its accuracy, the fact that it provided a spatial distribution of plant biomass, and it reduced labour requirements by eliminating the 1 day per week needed to monitor pastures.

In a survey of 63 primary producers on the usefulness of the technology in 2002 (Sneddon J.N., *pers. comm.*), the potential values identified were:
1. 82 % indicated increased confidence in making pasture and stock management decisions
2. 61% believed it helped them better manage risk
2. 59% stated it contributed to increased profitability
3. 34% indicated it saved time and effort

These findings are consistent with previous studies (Sneddon & Mazzarol 2002) on the usefulness of the technology to farmers in southern Australia, where the perceived advantages lie in the accuracy of the data, the ability to substitute a time-consuming on-farm endeavour, and the ability to manage remotely.

Conclusions

The remote monitoring of estimated pasture biomass in paddocks, and its growth rate, provided in a cheap, accurate and timely manner, offers substantial potential to raise the productivity of the farm business. It is also possible that an objective measure of the spatial variation of pasture production will highlight opportunities to improve the environmental management of the landscape, with areas of low performance either being corrected or retired to activities that have environmental benefit.

The relative advantage of the technology is likely to be realised by driving down enterprise costs and increasing output value. Market research (Sneddon & Mazzarol 2002) has indicated that farmers whose enterprises are highly sensitive to external forces are more likely to respond by adopting innovative grazing practices to maximise pasture utilisation (as these technologies have the potential to reduce perceived production and environmental risk). According to Swinton and Lowenberg-DeBoer (2002) Australia has the right mix of labour scarcity and abundance of land to make remotely sensed and precision agriculture technologies attractive and viable. They predict that there will be rapid adoption of these technologies in Australia, Canada and USA. Lessons learnt from precision agriculture in the cropping industry are that systems that are developed must meet the needs of the user in terms of their capital outlay, ease of use and compatibility with existing farming systems.

The provision of pasture forecasts meeting these criteria is a prime focus of our current research. At June 2000, 58% of Australian farms used a computer (17% increase on March 1999) and 34% used the Internet, a 91% increase on March 1999 (ABS, 2000). Australian farmers are adopting the Internet faster than any other industry or household group, providing an appropriate route for dissemination of pasture information. The future farm may well combine these pasture measurements with electronic systems to monitor animal performance and control access to feed.

References

ABS. 2000. Use of information technology on farms, Australia: 6. Canberra: Australian Bureau of Statistics.

Cayley, J. W. D. and Bird, P. R. 1996. Techniques for measuring pastures. Pastoral and Veterinary Institute, Hamilton, Victoria, Australia.

Edirisinghe, A., Hill, M, J., Donald, G.E., Hyder, M., Warren, B., Wheaton, G.A., and Smith, R.C.G. 2000. "Estimation of Feed on Offer and Growth Rate of Pastures using remote Sensing", 10th Australian Remote Sensing and Photogrammetry Conference, paper No. 112, Adelaide, Australia.

Edirisinghe. A, Donald, G.E., Hill, M.J. and Henry, D. 2002. "Precision management of feed supply through delivery of biomass and growth rate estimates of Western Australian annual pastures", 29th International Symposium on Remote Sensing of Environment, Buenos Aires, Argentina.

Haydock, K. P. and Shaw, N. H. 1975. The comparative method for estimating dry matter yield of pasture. Australian Journal of Experimental Agriculture and Animal Husbandry 15 663-670.

Henry, D.A., Edirisinghe, A., Donald, G. and Hill, M. 2002. Monitoring pastures using satellite remote sensing. Proceedings of the Australian Society of Animal Production 24 81-84.

House, R., Bilney, R., Ladyman, D., Oldham, C.M., Pagononi, B. and Yelland, M. 2002. Producing wool to budget using the 'Measure and you grow' approach - wool producer experience. Proceedings of the Australian Society of Animal Production 24 101-104.

Michael, P.J., Grimm, M., Hyder, M.W., Doyle, P.T. and Mangano, G.P. 1997. 'The effects of pasture pest damage and grazing management on efficiency of animal production'. MRC Final Report DAW 048.

Oldham, C.M., Gherardi, S.G., Paganoni, B. and Yelland, M. 2002. A new approach to managing wool production 'Measure as you grow'. Proceedings of the Australian Society of Animal Production 24 161-164.

Sneddon, J.N., Mazzarol, T. and Souter, G. 2000. A Feasibility Study of the Commercial Delivery of remotely Sensed Pasture Management Information. Perth, Graduate School of Management, University of Western Australia: 25pp.

Sneddon, J.N. and Mazzarol, T. 2002. Marketing approach critical to the diffusion of remotely sensed pasture management technologies. Proceedings of the Australian Society of Animal Production 24 221-224.

Swinton, S.M. and Lowenberg-DeBoer, J. 2002. Global adoption of precision agriculture technologies: Electronic source: Online University Discussion Paper, Michigan State and Purdue Universities.

Thompson, A.N., Hyder, M.W. and Doyle, P.T. 1997. Effects of differential grazing of annual pastures in spring and age of sheep on pasture and sheep production. Australian Journal of Experimental Agriculture 37 727-736.

Acknowledgements

We wish to acknowledge the skilled contribution made by staff of the Department of Agriculture WA, the team of the Satellite Remote Sensing Services of the Department of Land Administration WA, and colleagues in CSIRO.

Improving oestrus detection in dairy cows by combination of different traits using fuzzy logic

J. Krieter, R. Firk, E. Stamer and W. Junge
Institut für Tierzucht und Tierhaltung der Christian-Albrechts-Universität, 24118 Kiel, Herman-Rodewaldstr. 6, Germany
jkrieter@tierzucht.uni-kiel.de

Abstract

The present study investigates oestrus detection in dairy cows using serial data from management information systems. Data recording was performed on a commercial farm (n=862 cows). Activity, milk yield, milk flow rate and electrical conductivity were recorded automatically during each milking period. Additional information about previous oestrus (time interval since last oestrus) was available for 373 cows. Oestrus detection (day of insemination) was based on time series consisting of 15 days before and 15 days after oestrus. The univariate analyses were performed by different smoothing methods (day-to-day comparison, moving average, exponential smoothing). For multivariate analyses a fuzzy logic model was developed. The efficiency of the different models was determined by the parameters sensitivity and error rate.

The comparison between smoothing methods resulted in moderate differences for the different traits. Using the trait activity, sensitivity ranged between 94.2 and 71.0% and error rate was between 53.2 and 21.5% for threshold values between 40 and 120%. Milk yield, milk flow rate and conductivity were not suitable for improving oestrus detection. By considering activity and previous information in a multivariate fuzzy logic model sensitivity was 88.9% and error rate was reduced to 23.8%.

Keywords: oestrus detection, smoothing methods, multivariate analysis, fuzzy logic

Introduction

Undetected and falsely detected oestrus results in missed and untimely inseminations with consequent losses of income. One replicated insemination results in costs of 76.7 Euro (Hühn and Wähner, 1998). As calculated by Mack (1996) a one-day-prolonged calving interval induces costs of 0.6 to 1.2 Euro per cow.

In the present study, suitability of activity, milk yield, milk flow rate, electrical conductivity and information about previous oestrus cases for automatic oestrus detection in field data were analysed. In a first step the traits were analysed in an univariate manner, secondly the additional gain in oestrus detection was investigated if the traits were analysed multivariately by using fuzzy logic.

Material and methods

Collection of data was performed on a commercial dairy farm from February to December 1998. During this period approx. 50,000 observations of activity, milk yield, milk flow rate and electrical conductivity from 862 Holstein Friesian cows were accumulated. Activity was measured by pedometer, which was attached to the left foreleg of each cow. Milk yield, milk flow rate, electrical conductivity and activity were recorded at each milking in the milking parlour. All the traits were expressed on a daily basis according to Firk (2002). The parameter 'period since last oestrus' includes information about previous inseminations and previous oestrus cases. For each day considered in the analysis the period since last oestrus was calculated from the difference between the actual day and the day of previous information. Previous information was available for 373 cows.

The day of oestrus was determined by an insemination, which was followed by a calving after 265 to 295 days. This insemination was the only date on which the cow was certainly in oestrus. For oestrus detection, time series consisting of 15 days before oestrus, the day of oestrus and 15 days after oestrus were analysed. Due to missing values, the number of cows with complete time series differed between traits (table 1).

Table 1. Number of cows with complete time series, number of milkings, mean values (mean) and standard deviations (s.d.) for the trait activity, milk yield, milk flow rate and electrical conductivity.

Trait	Unit	Number of cows	Number of milkings	mean	s.d.
Activity	connections/h	862	54,740	4.4	2.9
Milk yield	kg	838	54,503	13.1	2.2
Milk flow rate	kg/min	663	41,895	2.2	0.5
Electrical conductivity	ms/cm	836	54,416	493.8	50.6

The automatic analysing of single data (univariate analyses) was realised by application of a day-to-day comparison, a moving average and an exponential smoothing based on previously applied smoothing methods for oestrus or mastitis detection (Arney et al., 1994; Yang, 1998; Secchiari et al., 1999). The purpose of smoothing methods is to calculate a forecast value ($\hat{Y}_{N+1}$) on the basis of previous observation values (Y_N) for each trait. If the relative deviation between $\hat{Y}_{N+1}$ and Y_N exceeded a given threshold, the cow was reported in oestrus.

By use of a day-to-day comparison the current measurement is compared with the measurement of the previous milking or day, respectively.

$$\hat{Y}_{N+1} = Y_N \qquad (1)$$

The comparison value of a moving average consists of a running mean out of a defined amount of previous observations for the same cow (Mottram, 1997).

$$\hat{Y}_{N+1} = \sum_{t=1}^{N} Y_t / N \qquad (2)$$

The smoothing effect of the moving average increases with the increasing number of considered observations in history. Analyses for all traits were performed with 5 and 10 values in history, respectively.

The exponential smoothing represents a special form of a moving average. Different weights can be given to previous observations (Secchiari et al., 1999).

$$\hat{Y}_{N+1} = \sum_{t=0}^{N} \alpha \cdot (1-\alpha)^t \cdot Y_{N-t} \qquad \text{with } \alpha=0.2, 0.4, 0.6, 0.8 \qquad (3)$$

The chosen α-value decreases exponentially with increasing distance between history value and actual observation, for high α-values stronger than for low α-values.

An improvement in oestrus detection was expected by multivariate analyses of the traits. The combination of traits was realised by fuzzy logic models, which were derived with Matlab (2000). Essential elements of a fuzzy model are the fuzzification, fuzzy inference and defuzzification (for a detailed description s. Altrock, 1995; Yang, 1998; Firk, 2002).

In contrast to common sets, where each element belongs to a set or not, fuzzy sets have a range of memberships between 0 and 1, each element can belong to special degrees and to several sets (fuzzification). Figure 1 illustrates an example of the shape of the membership functions 'short', 'normal', 'longish' and 'long' of the trait period since last oestrus. The results of fuzzification are the degrees of membership. For example, a period of 19 days since last oestrus would result in a degree of membership of 0.25 for the membership function 'short' and 0.75 for the membership 'normal'. The degrees of membership for the membership functions 'longish' and 'long' would be 0. Corresponding fuzzy sets were implemented for all traits (Firk, 2002).

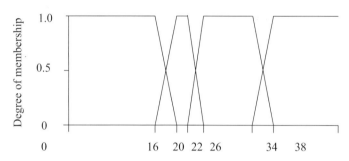

Figure 1. Membership functions for trait period since last oestrus (days).

The results from fuzzification present the input values for the fuzzy inference, the membership functions of one trait were combined with the membership functions of the other traits using the form: if condition, then conclusion. For each combination a conclusion was drawn regarding the incidence of oestrus, e.g. if activity is middle and milk flow rate is low then the cow is in oestrus. The reduction of the degrees of membership to one value per rule was realised by application of the operators Max and Min, which was used as input for the defuzzification.

In defuzzification, fuzzy values were transformed back into crisp results. The degrees of membership determined special areas below the membership functions 'not in oestrus' and 'in oestrus'. These areas were added and the result of defuzzification was calculated by application of the method centre of gravity. Values equal or higher than 0.5 were treated as oestrus warnings. Methods and traits were evaluated using the classification into correctly detected oestrus (true positives, TP) and observations outside oestrus periods (true negatives, TN). The degree of misclassification was expressed by false positive (FP) and false negative (FN) events. Sensitivity (SE) and error rate (ER) were calculated from these figures. The sensitivity indicated the probability of correctly classified oestrus on all oestrus cases (SE=TP/[TP+FN]), the number of false oestrus warnings in relation to the number of detected oestrus was expressed by the parameter error rate (ER=FP/[FP+TP]).

Results and discussion

The univariate analyses were performed to investigate the potential benefit of the traits activity, milk yield, milk flow rate and electrical conductivity for oestrus detection. In addition, for each trait a comparison between the time series methods day-to-day comparison, moving average and exponential smoothing was performed. Except for the day-to-day comparison, analyses were performed with varying observations in the history of the time series methods. The optimal size of history was 10 values for analysing the trait activity. Best results for oestrus detection based on the traits milk yield, milk flow rate and electrical conductivity were achieved by histories of 5 values of the time series methods. The following results are based on the optimal size of history for each time series method and trait. Results for oestrus detection by the trait activity are presented in figure 2.

The sensitivity decreased with increasing threshold value with a similar gradient for the analysed time series methods. Independent of the threshold value, the best results for sensitivity were achieved by a moving average with 94.2 to 71.0%. Lowest sensitivities were calculated by the day-to-day comparison with 93.5 and 61.5%.

The error rate decreases with increasing threshold value. Lowest error rates resulted from oestrus detection by moving average with a history of 10 values with 53.2 to 21.5%. Results for the exponential smoothing with a history of 10 values and a (-value of 0.4 were on the same level (53.4 to 23.1%). Maatje et al. (1997) calculated for a threshold of 100% a comparable sensitivity, with 78%, but the corresponding error rate was higher (32%). Mele et al. were able to detect 86.6% cows of all cows in oestrus, but 48.3% of oestrus warnings were false.

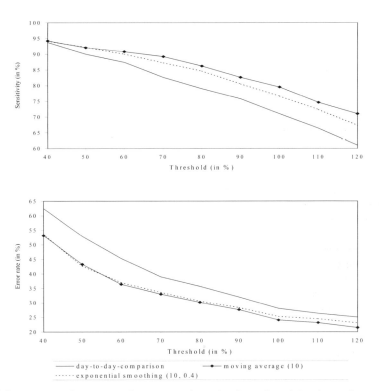

Figure 2. Sensitivity and error rate for oestrus detection by trait activity, depending on threshold and on forecasting method (n=862 cows).

For oestrus detection by the traits milk yield, milk flow rate and electrical conductivity only small differences in sensitivity and error rate between the time series methods occurred. The sensitivities and error rates were calculated by the best suited time series method for each trait (table 2). Low threshold values resulted in high sensitivities for all traits. A threshold value of 10% resulted in low sensitivities for electrical conductivity and milk yield, with 52.8 and 31.6% respectively, and moderate sensitivity for milk flow rate with 90.2%. Independent of threshold value, the error rate was high for all traits with 96.0 to 91.7%. As reported by Schofield (1989), milk yield and milk flow rate are not significantly affected by oestrus. Yang (1998) confirmed that variation in milk yield was not very pronounced due to oestrus.

The combination of activity with milk traits did not improve the results for oestrus detection (table 3). Independent of the combined traits, the parameter sensitivity and error rate both decreased. The simultaneous consideration of activity and all milk traits resulted in a sensitivity of 87.2% and an

Table 2. Sensitivity (%) and error rate (%) for oestrus detection by different traits and threshold values (%), calculated with the best suited smoothing methods.

Trait	Threshold	Sensitivity	Error rate
Activity[1]	60	90.8	36.4
	80	86.2	30.2
	100	79.5	24.1
Conductivity[2]	3	98.2	96.0
	10	52.8	94.2
Milk flow[3]	3	99.5	95.6
	10	90.2	93.8
Milk yield[4]	3	90.7	95.2
	10	31.6	91.7

1) n=862 cows; moving average with 10 values; 2) n=836 cows; exponential smoothing, with 5 values and an α value of 0.4; 3) n=663 cows; exponential smoothing, with 5 values and an α value of 0.4; 4) n=838 cows; day-to-day comparison

Table 3. Sensitivity (%) and error rate (%) for oestrus detection by different combinations of traits using fuzzy logic (n=862 cows).

Trait 1	Trait 2	Trait 3	Trait 4	Sensitivity	Error rate
Activity	Milk yield			87.6	30.1
Activity	Flow rate			87.0	29.2
Activity	Conductivity			87.4	31.0
Activity	Milk yield	Flow rate		87.9	29.1
Activity	Milk yield	Conductivity		87.4	29.7
Activity	Flow rate	Conductivity		87.7	29.0
Activity	Milk yield	Flow rate	Conductivity	87.2	28.2
Activity	Period[1]			88.9	23.8
Activity	Period[2]			87.9	12.5

1)period since last oestrus; 2)only cows with information about previous oestrus (n=373 cows)

error rate of 28.2%. Including previous oestrus information improved oestrus detection. Despite the decrease in sensitivity for the multivariate model with 373 cows to 87.9% (cows with information about previous oestrus), an obvious improvement in oestrus detection was realised due to a strong reduction in false positive oestrus warnings (ER=12.5%). These results were different to the results of De Mol and Woldt (2001), who could not found an improvement in oestrus detection by considering previous oestrus information. The authors calculated sensitivities between 73 and 79% and specificities between 98.1 and 98.8%. The simultaneous analysis of cows with and without previous oestrus information led to an increase in error rate to 23.8%, indicating the high number of cows without previous oestrus recording. Simultaneously, the sensitivity improved to 88.9%.

Conclusion

The univariate analysis of the trait activity resulted in satisfying results for sensitivity with 94.2 to 71.0% depending on threshold value. The corresponding error rate were high with 53.2 to 21.5%. The traits milk yield, milk flow rate and conductivity yielded no additional gain in oestrus detection. The fuzzy logic model gave a major improvement in detection results using activity and period since last oestrus. The number of false positives events was much lower. The combination of the smoothing models for the calculation of the deviation between predicted and actual values with the fuzzy logic model for the classification of these deviations gave a detection method of practical interest.

References

Altrock, C. 1995. Fuzzy Logic, Band 1, Technologie. R. Oldenbourg Verlag.

Arney, D.R., Kitwood, S.E., Philipps, C.J.C. 1994. The increase in activity during oestrus in dairy cows. Appl. Anim. Behav. Sci. 40, 211-218.

De Mol, R.M., Woldt, W.E. 2001. Application of fuzzy logic in automated cow status monitoring. J. Dairy Sci. 84, 400-410.

Firk, R. 2002. Methods and traits for automatic oestrus detection in dairy cows. Schriftenreihe des Instituts für Tierzucht und Tierhaltung der Christian-Albrechts-Universität, Kiel, Heft 130.

Hühn, U., Wähner, M. 1998. Ökonomische Bewertung der Brunstsynchronisation bei Rind und Schwein. In: Fruchtbarkeitsmanagement bei Rind und Schwein. Hrsg. Arbeitskreis Großtierpraxis, VAV, Verl. für Agrarwiss. und Veterinärmedizin, 1998.

Maatje, K., Loeffler, S.H., Engel, B. 1997. Predicting optimal time of insemination in cows that show visual signs of oestrus by estimating onset of oestrus with pedometer. J. Dairy Sci. 80, 1098-1105.

Mack, G. 1996. Wirtschaftlichkeit des züchterischen Fortschritts in Milchviehherden - Gesamtbetriebliche Analyse mit Hilfe eines simultan-dynamischen linearen Planungsansatzes. Ph.D. Thesis. University of Hohenheim, Germany.

Matlab 2000. The MathWorks, Inc., Version 6.0.0.88.

Mele, M., Secchiari, P., Serra, A., Ferruzzi, G., Paoletti, F., Biagioni, M. 2001. Application of the 'tracking signal' method to the monitoring of udder health and oestrus in dairy cows. Livest. Prod. Sci. 72, 279-284.

Mottram, T. 1997. Automatic monitoring of the health and metabolic status of dairy cows. Livest. Prod. Sci. 48, 209-217.

Schofield, S.A. 1989. Oestrus detection methods and oestrus behaviour of dairy cows in different environments. Dissertation Abstracts International B, Science and Engineering, 49 :7, 2432.

Secchiari, P., Mele, M., Leotta, R. 1999. An exponential smoothing model in time series analysis of milk electrical conductivity data for the clinical mastitis detection. 50th Anual Meeting of the European Association of Animal Production Zurich, Switzerland 23-26 August 1999.

Yang,Y. 1998. Rechnergestützte Östrusüberwachung bei Milchkühen unter Anwendung der Fuzzy Logic Methode. Ph.D. Thesis, University of Munich, Germany.

Telemetric measurement of heart rate and heart rate variability for evaluating psychological stress induced by visual discrimination learning in dwarf goats

J. Langbein[1], G. Nürnberg[2] and G. Manteuffel[1]
[1]Research Institute for the Biology of Farm Animals, Division Behavioural Physiology, Wilhelm-Stahl-Allee 2, D-18196 Dummerstorf, Germany
[2]Research Institute for the Biology of Farm Animals, Division Genetics & Biometry, Wilhelm-Stahl-Allee 2, D-18196 Dummerstorf, Germany
langbein@fbn-dummerstorf.de

Abstract

We studied visual discrimination learning in dwarf goats using a computer based learning device. Varying visual stimuli were presented on a computer screen in a four-choice design. To get a reward goats had to choose the correct stimulus by pressing a button next to the correct stimulus. To evaluate psychological stress with regard to learning success we analysed non-invasively measured heart rate (HR) and heart rate variability (HRV). Ten animals out of twelve reached a stable level of correct choice of above 70 % at the end of three consecutive learning tasks. Whereas HR increased significantly throughout task one, this relationship was inverted in tasks two and three, indicating different coping strategies with regard to the coping predictability concept. Results of HRV suggested changes in HR related to psychological stress during learning resulting from alterations of the vago-sympathetic balance predominantly caused by a withdrawal of vagal control of the heart.

Keywords: learning, psychological stress, heart rate variability, vagal control

Introduction

The number of published studies which use operant learning techniques in farm animals is rapidly increasing (Kilgour et al, 1991). This approach has been applied at first to investigate their sensory capacities (Arave, 1996) and latterly to study general aspects of learning in farm animals (Nicol, 1996). This is all the more important in the context of an increased level of automation and advanced self-management systems in actual animal husbandry. Knowledge about farm animal cognition is currently attracting further research in the field of suffering in animals resulting from psychological under-demanding under boring husbandry conditions (Sneddon et al., 2000). Fundamental research on learning which has largely been the preserve of experimental psychologists is also interested in showing how mental effort related to learning acts as a stressor itself as well as how stress interferes with learning success. To evaluate husbandry systems with regard to animal welfare it is important to know what learning means to animals related to stress. Therefore the aims of this project were to study learning capacities of dwarf goats and stress induced by learning in visual discrimination tasks. To assess changes in the vago-sympathetic balance related to psychological stress we analysed telemetrically measured heart rate (HR) and heart rate variability (HRV) at various levels of learning effort and success (Sharpley et al, 2002).

Animals, materials and methods

Learning device and learning tasks

In order to examine visual learning in dwarf goats we employed three visual discrimination tasks. We tested a group of 12 young males from 15 to 22 weeks of age using a computer based learning device integrated in the home pen of the animals (Figure 1A). To get a small amount of water (30 ml) animals had to press one of four buttons in front of a 14" computer monitor about 15 to 35 cm above a waterer. Each of the buttons was arranged next to a segment of the monitor (Figure 1B). Animals wore transponders for time related registration of all actions of individuals at the buttons. All goats were first trained to press reliably on all buttons in front of the monitor to get water over a period of six weeks (adaptation period). Following learning tasks lasted for thirteen days each. In every task four visual stimuli were presented on a computer screen in a four-choice design (Figure 1C). The visual stimuli were designed to be more complex with each ensuing task. To get water as a reward goats had to choose the correct stimulus by pushing the button next to the monitor segment the stimulus was presented on. The same stimuli were presented in a distinct pattern following a quasi random series. We analysed individual learning success on a daily basis. For reasons of animal welfare we separately supervised the number of correct choices per day per animal to be sure all animals got the daily water amount they needed.

Heart beat measurements

The device system Polar S810 (®Polar Elektro Oy, Finland) was used for telemetric measurement of heartbeat activity (R-R interval). For technical description and details of its application in farm animals see Mohr et al (2002). Goats were adapted to the measuring equipment in the last two weeks of the adaptation period. Measurements of HR and HRV were done during the last two days

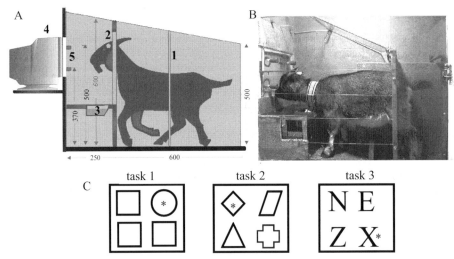

Figure 1. A. Drawing and measures of the box with the learning device: 1 = aerial for animal identification, 2 = yoke to put the head through, 3 = waterer, 4 = computer screen for presenting visual stimuli, 5 = press buttons to choose a stimulus. 1 B. Snapshot of a dwarf goat acting at the learning device. 1 C. Visual stimuli used in the three consecutive learning tasks (* = correct stimulus, S^+).

of the adaptation period as well as at the beginning (day 1, 2) and at the end (day 12, 13) of each learning task. Every day we measured six animals at the same time, from 08:00 to 11:00 and from 13:00 to 16:00. Only such parts of the tachograms which were recorded when animals were laying down without external disturbances, lasted at least 10 minutes and had a corrected fault rate of less than 10 percent were included in the analysis. HR and HRV parameters in the time domain (SDNN = square root of variance of all R-R intervals, RMSSD = root mean square of successive differences of R-R intervals), and in the frequency domain (LF_{norm} = normalized power of the low-frequency band, HF_{norm} = normalized power of the high-frequency band) were calculated from a gliding 5 min window which was moving over the data set with a temporal shift of 150 sec (for detailed description see Mohr et al, 2002). Calculation of HRV parameters was done using the MULTIDAT computer program (© by Mohr, 1997).

Statistical analyses

Three statistical models were used for data analysis. At first repeatedly measured data on learning success within the three learning tasks, sampled over 13 test days each, were analysed by a mixed model, with two fixed effects (learning task and test day), a random factor animal and corresponding interactions. Effects of the learning task and the period within the task (beginning or end) on HR and HRV parameters were analysed using the same mixed linear model with two fixed effects (learning task and period within the task) and again a random factor animal and corresponding interactions. Post-hoc tests between tasks at single days in the first model and between the periods within each task in the second model were calculated using the Tukey-Cramer correction, to ensure a multiple test risk of first kind ≤ 0.05. A third model, for a comparison between the adaptation period and the single learning tasks, was done separately for beginning period and end period using the Dunnett-Hsu test (adjusted). For all three models we used the procedure MIXED of SAS© (SAS Systems, Release 8.2, SAS Institute Inc., Cary, NC).

Results

Learning success

Learning success in the three different visual discrimination tasks is presented in figure 2. We analysed data of only ten animals because two individuals did not learn any of the stimuli at all. The mixed linear model revealed a significant influence of the task as well as of the test day. Learning success started at a level of correct choice below 25 % (level of chance) in task one. Animals reached a stable level of correct choice of about 70 % not before day ten. The learning curve follows the sigmoid type. In contrast, in tasks two and three learning success started at a level of 45 %, and animals reached a level of correct choice of approximately 70 % already at day six. The learning curves seemed quite similar in both of these tasks and followed the logarithmic type. No differences in learning success were found between these two tasks. Differences in learning success were significant between task one and task two and three throughout day one to day nine.

Heart rate

Changes in the HR throughout all measuring periods are given in figure 3. We found a significant influence of the task as well as of task * period (beginning/end). Whereas the HR was significantly higher at the end of task one compared to the beginning, this ratio was inverted in task two and task three ($p ≤ 0.05$) when the HR declined from the beginning to the end. Compared to the adaptation period the HR was significantly higher at the beginning of task two and significantly lower at the end of task three.

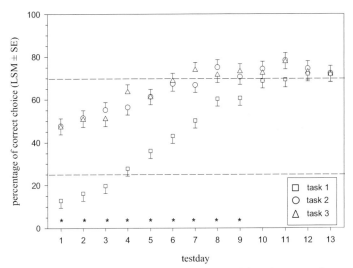

Figure 2. Least square means (± SE) of learning success of dwarf goats in three consecutive visual discrimination tasks (n = 10). Lower dashed line indicates level of chance, upper line indicates a level of correct choice of 70 %. Asterisks below the curves mark significant differences between task one and the following two tasks. No differences were found between task two and task three.

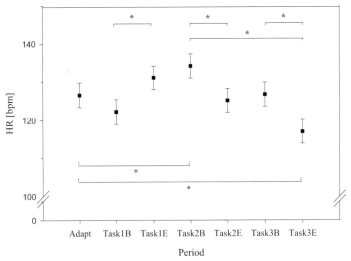

Figure 3. Least square means (± SE) of the HR of dwarf goats in the adaptation period and throughout three visual discrimination tasks (Adapt = Adaptation, B = beginning, E = end; n = 10). Significant differences between periods within learning tasks (above the graph) as well as between adaptation period and learning tasks (below the graph) are indicated.

Precision lifestock farming

Heart rate variability

Concerning HRV we found a significant influence of the task as well as of task * period (beginning/end) on the RMSSD, on the ratio RMSSD/SDNN indicating changes in the vago-sympathetic balance and on the HF_{norm}. Testing differences between the periods within each task and between tasks only the ratio RMSSD/SDNN showed significant changes inversely related to changes of the HR (figure 4). When analysing differences between the adaptation period and the learning tasks, separately for the beginning and the end, we found a significant effect of the model on the RMSSD, the ratio of RMSSD/SDNN and on the HF_{norm} at the beginning and on the ratio RMSSD/SDNN at the end. However, when comparing differences between single periods only the ratio RMSSD/SDNN was lower at the beginning of task two compared to the adaptation period.

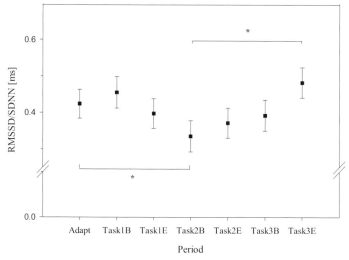

Figure 4. Least square means (± SE) of the Ratio RMSSD/SDNN in the adaptation period and throughout three visual discrimination tasks (n = 10). Significant differences between periods within learning tasks (above the graph) as well as between adaptation and learning tasks (below the graph) are indicated.

Discussion

We studied visual discrimination learning in dwarf goats using a computer based learning device integrated in the home pen of the animals (Franz et al, 2002). In so doing, in contrast to classical learning experiments, animals themselves decided when to visit the learning box. Results show the capability of dwarf goats for successful visual discrimination learning in a self-controlled group learning design (Soltysik & Baldwin, 1972, Baldwin, 1979). The course of the learning curves was basically different in task one compared to the following two tasks. Despite a six week adaptation period to the learning device with positive reinforcement shaping of the button pressing response the animals had to adopt to the discrimination task itself during task one. In terms of learning theory at least the first days of this task one may be looked upon as part of the shaping procedure. When reaching a level of correct choice of about 70 % the learning curve flattened indicating a slowdown of learning motivation accompanied by a constant rate of errors throughout the day. Learning success far above the level of chance was achieved already at day one in task two and three indicating very fast learning during the first visits of the learning box when animals were familiar with the discrimination task. In accordance with task one learning motivation stagnated when reaching a level of correct choice of 70 %. No differences between learning curves in task two and three demonstrate that the goats are capable of discriminating similarly between closed and open shapes (Baldwin, 1979).

To evaluate the level of stress with regard to the learning process we analysed HR and HRV only from measurements of resting animals to exclude influences of physical activity on these parameters. In doing so, we did not evaluate acute mental stress during the learning process itself but the level of psychological stress caused by a lower or higher effort demanded from the animals to get water depending on learning success. In terms of stress physiology, reverse change of HR in task one compared to the following two tasks suggested a different level of psychological stress and accordingly different coping strategies depending on the novelty of the task. With regard to the coping predictability concept by Henry & Stephens (1977), loss of control over drinking water at the beginning of task one seemed to provoke a certain level of frustration in the animals because of uncontrollable stimuli (decrease of HR). This fits the simultaneous stagnation of learning success during the first days of task one (shaping). An increase of HR (indicating higher level of arousal) were not seen before the animals established an association between visual stimuli, press button and the water reward. Even at the end of task one animals still intensively dealt with the learning situation as the high level of HR indicated. In contrast, when animals were familiar with the procedure in tasks two and three, increased HR at the beginning implies active coping right from the start of the tasks (learning) and led to a reduced level of stress with increased learning success at the end.

Analysis of HRV enables detailed analyses which branch of the autonomic nervous system (ANS) mediated the effect of a psychological stressor on the heart both under normal conditions and in reaction to external stressors (Pagani et al, 1995). Horses in a novel object test showed a marked shift of the balance of the ANS towards sympathetic dominance, presumably related to vagal withdrawal while simultaneous sympathetic activation (Visser et al, 2002). Studying the impact of psychological stress on the cardiovascular system of rats Sgoifo et al (1997, 1999) concluded that changes in HR during social defeat cannot be explained simply in terms of higher sympathetic activity to the heart, but also in terms of a concomitant lack of vagal rebound to sympathetic activation. However these studies analysed heart rate of active animals when vagal tone is already reduced. Results presented in this study, done on resting animals, suggested that changes of HR related to psychological stress for the most part are caused by a withdrawal of the vagal tone at the heart. We found significant influences of the single task as well as of the period within the task on HRV parameters which indicate changes of vagal activity at the heart (RMSSD, RMSSD/SDNN, HF_{norm}). At the same time, HRV parameters which at least partly reflect also modulations of the sympathetic activity like SDNN and LF_{norm} did not show any significant changes. These results are in agreement with the polyvagal theory by Porges (1995, 2001) who considered a special myelinated branch of the nervous vagus originating from the nucleus ambiguus as a main mediator in reaction to psychological stress.

References

Arave, C.W. 1996. Assessing sensory capacity of animals using operant technology. J Anim Sci 74 1996-2009.

Baldwin, B.A. 1979. Operant studies on shape discrimination in goats. Physiology & Behavior 23 455-459.

Franz, H., Roitberg, E., Löhrke, B., Nürnberg, G., Dietl, G. and Kinzelbach, R. 2002. Visual discrimination learning of group-housed goats at an automated learning device. Arch Tierz 4 387-401.

Henry, J.P. and Stephens, P.M. 1977. Stress, health and the social environment. A sociobiologic approach to medicine. Spinger Verlag, New York.

Kilgour, R., Foster, T.M., Temple, W., Matthews, L.R. and Bremner, K.J. 1991. Operant technology applied to solving farm animal problems. An assessment. Appl Anim Behav Sci 30 141-166.

Mohr, E., Langbein, J. and Nürnberg, G. 2002. Heart rate variability: An indicator of pathological and physiological stress in calves and cattle. Physiology & Behaviour 75 251-259.

Nicol, C.J. 1996. Farm animal cognition. Animal Science 62 375-391.

Pagani, M., Lucini, D., Rimoldi, O., Furlan, R., Piazza, S. and Biancardi, L. 1995. Effects of physical and mental exercise on heart rate variability. In: Malik, M. and Camm, A. (eds) Heart rate variability. Futura Publishing Company Inc., Armonk, pp 245-266.

Porges, S. W. 1995. Orienting in a defensive world: Mammalian modification of our evolutionary heritage. A polyvagal theory. Psychophysiology 32 301-318.

Porges, S.W. 2001. The polyvagal theory: phylogenetic substrates of a social nervous system. Int J Psychophysiol 42 123-146.

Sgoifo, A., De Boer, S.F., Westenbroek, C., Maes, F.W., Beldhuis, H., Suzuki, T. and Koolhaas, J.M. 1997. Incidence of arrhythmias and heart rate variability in wild-type rats exposed to social stress. Am. J. Physiol. 273 1754-1760.

Sgoifo, A., Koolhaas, J.M., Musso, E. and de Boer, S.F. 1999. Different sympathovagal modulation of heart rate during social and nonsocial stress episodes in wild-type rats. Physiology & Behavior 67 733-738.

Sharpley, C.S., Kamen, P., Galatsis, M., Heppel, R., Veivers, C. and Claus, K. 2000. An Examination of the Relationship Between Resting Heart Rate Variability and Heart Rate Reactivity to a Mental Arithmetic Stressor. Appl Psychophysiology and Biofeedback 25 143-154.

Sneddon, I.A., Beattie, V.E., Dunne, L. and Neil, W. 2000. The effect of environmental enrichment on learning in pigs. Animal welfare 9 359-372.

Soltysik, S. and Baldwin, B.A. 1972. The performance of goats in triple choice delayed response tasks. Acta Neurobiol Exp (Warsz) 32 73-86.

Visser, E.K., van Reenen, C.G., van der Werf, J.T.N., Schilder, M.B.H., Knaap, J.H., Barneveld, A. and Blokhuis, A.J. 2002. Heart rate and heart rate variability during a novel object test and a handling test in young horses. Physiology & Behavior 76 289-296.

Acknowledgement

The authors are grateful to Miss K. Siebert and Mr. D. Sehland for assisting with data recording, data management and technical support at all phases of the experiments. We want to thank E. Mohr for offering the MULTIDAT program for data analysis and two referees for their comments, which improved the manuscript. We are also grateful to Martina Kretschmer for reviewing the English.

Variable milking frequency in large dairies: performance and economic analysis - models and experiments

E. Maltz[1], N. Livshin[1], A. Antler[1], Y. Edan[2], S. Matza[2] and A. Antman[3]

[1]*Institute of Agricultural Engineering, A.R.O., The Volcani Center, P.O. Box 6, Bet Dagan, 50250, Israel*

[2]*Department of Industrial Engineering and Management, Faculty of Engineering Sciences, Ben-Gurion University of the Negev, Beer Sheva 84105, Israel*

[3]*Ma'agan-Yonatan Dairy, Yonatan, 12415, Israel*

emaltz@volcani.agri.gov.il

Abstract

In Israel, 20% of the monthly production quota that is "shifted" from winter to summer gets a bonus of 26.5% for each "shifted" kg. Variable milking frequency (MF) can be a tool to control milk yield (MY) to exploit these conditions. Dairies in which the milking parlor is operated most of the day, can milk different groups of cows at different MFs within the normal routine. However, manipulating MF is expected also to affect operational and food consumption costs, while not all cows will respond as expected. A study was undertaken to evaluate practically, economically, and physiologically the concept to suppress winter production of individually-selected cows that their economically-corrected-milk production (ECM) is lower than their MY, and encourage summer production individually-selected cows that their ECM is higher or equal to MY. The results indicated that manipulating MF to control production is feasible in large dairies. They were used to calibrate a pre-designed economic model that can help to economise production under varying market conditions.

Key words: Milking-frequency, large-dairies, milk yield control

Introduction

The dairy industry in Israel operates under an annual quota divided monthly and bound to seasonal supply and demand. It is permitted to transfer up to 20% of the quota from winter (January-May) to summer (July-November), with a bonus of 26.5% above the fixed price for every kg of milk shifted from winter to summer. In addition, the milk price policy in Israel favors milk with high protein and fat composition, and penalizes for milk volume (ECM = $-0.05*MY_{(kg)} + 8.8765*fat_{(kg)} + 26.628*protein_{(kg)}$). This leaves the manager with substantial operational freedom, but any management decision is affected by a variety of physiological variables (Grinspan et al. 1994, Maltz and Metz 1994, Maltz et al. 2002) which may produce unexpected results. So, the outcome of any management decision in the dairy industry is exposed to a great deal of uncertainty.

Increasing or decreasing MF influences MY (Hillerton et al. 1990, Ipema and Benders 1992) hence, be a tool to meet temporary constraints without taking drastic measures such as changing the number of cows, manipulation with drying off timing and reproduction strategy, or applying nutritional means. Changing MF is superior because of its simplicity and ability to go from constrained to enhanced production. This tool seems to be practical only in robotic milking dairies where cows in the same group can be milked in different MFs. Nevertheless, in large dairies, where the milking parlor is operated most of the day, it is possible to milk groups of cows with different MFs with minimal interference to daily milking parlor operations. For example, most of the cows can be milked three times daily while one or two groups can be milked twice or four times daily according to the specific economic goal. Decreasing MF from 3 to 2 times daily can be expected to reduce milk production by an average of about 10% (ICBA, 2001). Nevertheless, the response of different cows to a change in MF might differ according to their physiological capacity and ever-changing physiological status throughout lactation. Manipulating MF is expected to affect working hours, milking parlor operational cost, and food consumption that might impose additional costs on one hand, while not all cows will respond as expected on the other. Therefore, an optimal milking frequency policy should include a physiological and economic analysis of each cow in the herd to evaluate her ability to meet performance expectations while considering the economical benefits. Therefore, the relationships between MF, MY and composition are significant factors when selecting cows for reducing MF (depress MY) or increasing MF (encouraged MY). This paper evaluates the possibility to achieve the economic goal dictated by market forces by manipulating the MF of selected cows that are expected to respond physiologically in accordance to the economical goal. Another goal was to design a matching economic model based on economic and physiological assumptions and to be calibrated by experimental results.

Materials and methods

A dairy with 500-550 milking cows located in northern Israel was selected for testing the concept of variable MF. The 14X14 herringbone milking parlor is normally operated for 12-14 hours a day (including washing time) milking all cows three times daily at 03:30, 11:30, and 18:30. From mid April until end of June, an attempt was made to restrict production by reducing MF. All multiparous cows that were at least 60 days in milking and had an ECM/MY ratio lower than 1 were candidates for reducing MF. A 56 cows' lot was assigned to the cows milked twice daily because of available space and milking parlor capacity. There were no more than 80 cows which had an ECM/MY ratio less than 1. This prevented equal experiment and control groups. Therefore, the cows were clustered in groups of 3 according to: a) lactation number (2 or more), b) days in milk (DIM), and c) ECM/MY ratio. Two cows (randomly selected) of each cluster were assigned to twice-milking-a-day group (56 cows), and the third in her group served as control (28 cows). After ten weeks thrice daily milking was resumed. Cows whose MY was affected for any reason other than MF were excluded from the analysis. Because of an unusually large number of mastitis cases during this trial, we ended with 46 cows in the experimental group and 15 cows in the control group. The twice-daily MF group was milked last in the morning milking (at 07:00), and first in the evening milking (at 18:30). The milking intervals between the two milkings for this group were 11.5 and 12.5 hours. At the beginning of July an attempt was made to encourage production by increasing MF. We selected all pregnant cows that had an ECM/MY ratio of one or greater; were 150 DIM or more, and had a body weight (BW) of 500 kg or more and increasing. This time there were enough cows to create equal control and experiment groups. All cows were clustered in pairs (by criteria described above). One of each pair was randomly assigned to a 4 times daily milking group (intervals of 8, 4, 5, and 7 hours between milkings): the other was left in her group and served as a control. When a cow reached dry-off time, the pair was replaced by another one which resulted in a dynamic situation in the 4 times daily milked group. The cows were fed a flat rate total mixed ration (TMR) throughout the year according to NRC recommendations (NRC 2001). MY and BW were measured ($\pm$ 1% of actual value) daily by electronic milk meters, and walk through scales located in the outlet path from the milking parlor (S.A.E. Afikim, Afikim, Israel). The t-test was used for statistical analysis.

Using data from commercial farms in Israel we characterized normal MY production of multiparous cows into three periods: 60..120 DIM - no change in MY; 120..150 DIM - 5% decline. 150 DIM and greater - 10% decline.

The preliminary MY prediction model assumed a 10% reduction of MY for cows in which MF was reduced from 3 to 2 (ICBA, 2001). An economic analysis was conducted for one group of 112 cows (milking parlor consideration). All analysis was conducted on experiment data. To compare the two management strategies (thrice MF vs. variable MF) we initially assumed that the amount of milk that was not produced during the winter will be produced during the summer by: (1) Resumed thrice daily milking of cows that were restrained by twice milking daily during the winter. (2) by increasing milking frequency from 3 to 4 milkings a day for selected cows. The model takes into account three parameters: expected income, operational costs and food costs.

Results and discussion

Transfer from 3 to 2 milkings a day reduced MY after 10 weeks by about 10% more than the normal decline recorded in the control cows (Figures 1, 2). Most of which took place after one week (Figures 1, 2). However, while the MY decreased on average by 8.7 kg/cow during this period, ECM yield was reduced only by 4.2 kg/cow (Figure 1), only 6% more than that of the control cows (Figure 2). This was the result of milk composition improvement that accompanied the MY decline beyond the normal increase of milk solids along lactation (Table 1). After resuming thrice daily milking (week +1 Figures 1, 2) MY and ECM yield increased to levels similar to those of the cows that were milked thrice daily throughout. BW increased during the 10 weeks in both control and experiment cows (from an average of 614 kg to 636 kg (3.6%) and from 601 kg to 611 kg (1.7%) in the experiment ones respectively). The difference was statistically insignificant.

Transfer from 3 to 4 milkings a day improved lactation curve persistency (Figures 3, 4). This resulted in a lesser reduction in both MY (to 92.8% and 88.9% of pre-trial MY for experiment and control cows respectively, $P < 0.05$) and ECM yield (to 93% and 89.9% of pre-trial ECM for experiment and control cows respectively, $P < 0.1$). This was more evident in MY rather than ECM yield (Figures 3, 4) indicating a reverse correlation between MY and composition (Table 1).

BW increased similarly by about 5% of pre-trial weight (590 and 620 kg average weight for control and experiment cows respectively) during the 14 weeks.

The sensitivity analysis to the response for both decreased and increased MF showed that it correlates negatively with lactation number. The higher lactation the lower response. This means that variable MF frequency in large dairies can be improved beyond the results presented here by selecting the cows that respond best.

Table 1. Effect of reducing milking frequency from 2 to 3 (46 cows) and increasing from 3 to 4 (56 cows) on milk composition compared to cows milked 3 times daily.

	Before reducing milking frequency		10 week after reducing milking frequency	
	Milk fat %	Milk protein %	Milk fat %	Milk protein %
Cont	2.63	2.95	2.91	3.14
Exp	2.64	2.88	3.04*	3.06
	Before increasing milking frequency		After increasing milking frequency	
	Milk fat %	Milk protein %	Milk fat %	Milk protein %
Cont	3.77	3.32	3.80*	3.45*
Exp	3.55	3.31	3.62	3.52*

*Significant difference (P < 0.05) within group;

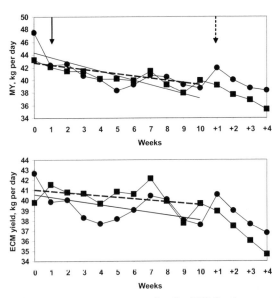

Figure 1. Milk yield (MY) and economic corrected milk (ECM) of cows milked 3 times daily (control ■) compared to cows transferred to 2 times milking (week 1 solid arrow) during 10 weeks, and resumed 3 times daily milking (week +1 broken arrow) (●). Broken line-trend line of control cows weeks 0-10, solid line-trend line of experiment cows.

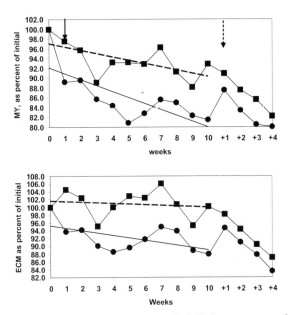

Figure 2. Milk yield (MY) and economic corrected milk (ECM) as percent of pretrial (week 0), of cows milked 3 times daily (control ■) compared to cows transferred to 2 times daily milking (week 1 solid arrow) during 10 weeks and resumed 3 times daily milking (week +1 broken arrow) (●). Broken line- trend line of control cows weeks 0-10, solid line - trend line of experiment cows weeks 0-10.

Precision lifestock farming

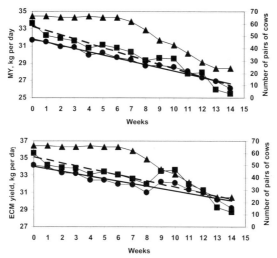

Figure 3. Milk yield (MY-upper panel) and economic corrected milk yield (ECM-lower panel) of cows milked 3 times daily (control ■) compared to experiment cows transferred to 4 times daily milking in week 1 during 14 weeks (●). Broken line- trend line of control cows, solid line-trend line of experiment cows. ▲- number of pairs of cows (exp, cont).

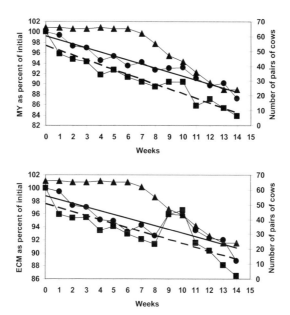

Figure 4. Milk yield (MY) and economically corrected milk yield (ECM) as percent of pretrial production (week 0), of cows milked 3 times daily (control ■) compared to experiment cows transferred to 4 times daily milking in week 1 during 14 weeks (●). Broken line- trend line of control cows, solid line - trend line of experiment cows. ▲- number of pairs (control and experiment) of cows.

The advantage of variable MF can be extended to any economic environment such as demand for milk proteins, when cows with superior milk composition can be milked more frequently while others with inferior composition are milked less frequently. In the large dairy higher and lower than thrice daily MF can be conducted simultaneously.

In respect of economic analysis, the milking parlor operated half an hour less during winter and the same time longer during the summer. An overall income increase of 4.2% would be expected if 10% of winter quota would have been produced during the summer. Practically, reduced MF of the cows selected in this trial caused a greater reduction than the capacity of the cows selected to increase production by increasing MF, probably because of over-cautiousness in selecting cows for high MF. Therefore, cows earlier in lactation and more first and second lactation cows have to be included.

Conclusions

Variable milking frequency can serve as a tool to control seasonal milk production to achieve an economic goal in a large dairy, through selection of physiologically fitted cows to which the variable MF is applied.

References

Grinspan, P., Kahn, H.E., Maltz, E. and Edan Y. 1994. A fuzzy logic expert system for dairy cow transfer between feeding groups. Transactions of the ASAE. (5):1647

Hillerton, J.E., Knight, C.H. Turvey, A. Wheatley, S.D. Wilde C.J. 1990. Milk yield and mammary function in dairy cows milked four times daily. J. Dairy Res. 57: 285-294.

ICBA, Israel Holstein Herdbook, 2001

Ipema, A.H., Benders, E. 1992. Production duration of machine milking and teat quality of dairy cows milked 2, 3, 4 times daily with variable intervals. Proc. Int. Symp Prospects for Automatic Milking. Wageningen, Netherlands, Ipema, A.H., Lippus, A.C., Metz, J.H.M., Rossing W. (eds). EAAP Publication. No. 65:244-252.

Maltz, E., Livshin, N., Devir, S. Rosenfeld. D. 2002. Using on-line data in management of milking frequency and concentrates supplementation in the AMS herd. Proc. of The First North American Conference on Robotic Milking, Toronto, Ontario, Canada, March 20-22, 2002:III 33-44.

Maltz, E. and Metz. J.H.M. 1994. An individual approach to manage the dairy cow: a challenge for research and practice. Proc. of International Symposium on Prospects for Future Dairying: A Challenge for Science and Industry. Lind, O. Svennersten K. (eds). Alfa Laval Agri, Tumba, Sweden and Swedish University of Agricultural Sciences, Uppsala, Sweden. 267-282.

National Research Council (NRC). 2001. Nutrition requirements of dairy cattle. Seventh revised edition, 2001. National Academic Press, Washington DC.

Evaluation of udder cleanliness by spectroscopy

D. Ordolff

Institut für Betriebstechnik und Bauforschung, FAL, D 38116 Braunschweig, Institut für Chemie und Technologie der Milch, BAfM, D 24103 Kiel, Germany
ordolff@bafm.de

Abstract

Analysis of spectroscopic parameters to evaluate the efficiency of cleaning udders and teats indicated that manual cleaning mainly caused modifications of reflectivity of surfaces. The parameters red/green and yellow/blue were not useful to indicate cleaning efficiency at white surfaces, but a significant reduction of the level of "yellow" due to cleaning was observed at black surfaces.

The parameter red/green was most efficient to detect bloodstained surfaces. Blood was present when a certain limit was exceeded.

A more practical evaluation of visual cleanliness is to be expected by the use of appropriate machine vision systems.

Keywords: Cleanliness, udder, teats, spectroscopy, reflected light.

Introduction

Automatic milking systems are not able to manage cleaning of udder and teats according to the demands of actual regulations, considering the actual status of cleanliness before and after cleaning procedures, and to detect lesions of teats.

Bull et al.(1995) did some basic research on application of optical parameters to fulfil these demands. Problems were mainly found with respect to pigmented surfaces. In a further step Bull et al. (1996) used images of a CCD-colour-camera to evaluate the cleanliness of teat surfaces. Connecting type and intensity of colours of all pixels resulted in correct recognition of dirty teats. False results only were observed at some clean teats. Mottram (1997) compared several types of dirty teat surfaces. Cleanliness of the barn and structure of faecal material were mainly affecting the condition of teat surfaces.

Based on experience with spectroscopic evaluation of foremilk (Ordolff, 2001) on the experimental station of the Federal Agricultural Research Centre (FAL) at Braunschweig it was investigated, to what extend spectroscopic industrial standards would be useful for evaluating the efficiency of cleaning teats and surrounding udder surfaces prior to milking in comparison to visual evaluation by milkers, responsible for correct manual cleaning.

Material and methods

In a first experiment in three milking sessions udder and teats of 76 cows were evaluated according to the standard CIE-lab, corresponding to DIN 6174, before and after being cleaned by a milker. Measurements were done using the spectroscopic measuring device SPECTROPEN (Manufacturer: Dr. Lange GmbH&Co. KG, Düsseldorf).

The data recording system applied uses three parameters to describe the optical condition of the evaluated surface. First, the level of reflected light (parameter L) is indicated by figures in the range from 0 to 100. Colours are paired to red/green (parameter a) and yellow/blue (parameter b). Neutral results are indicated by the value 0, positive or negative figures represent the level of dominance of individual colours.

In a further experiment the efficiency of the measuring device for detecting bloodstained surfaces was investigated. For this purpose spots of fresh blood were put on udders and teats of 13 cows. Six teats had dark surfaces. Colours were measured before and after manual cleaning.

For measuring the sensing device had to be brought in touch with the surface to be evaluated. The results obtained were processed according to type and cleaning status of each surface. For statistical treatments F-test and range-test according to Newman-Keuls (e.g. Haiger, 1966) were used.

Results and discussion

Surfaces before and after cleaning

White surfaces of udder and teats after cleaning reflected more light than before cleaning (Table 1). The amount of light reflected from teats with black surface generally was at a lower level and was even more reduced due to cleaning. The results obtained before and after cleaning in all cases were different at significant levels (P<1%).

Table 1. Reflectivity (L) of evaluated surfaces.

	Udder white		Teat white		Teat black	
	unclean	clean	unclean	clean	unclean	clean
n	23	23	34	34	19	19
Average	47,0	60,4	40,2	55,0	31,8	24,3
s	9,92	6,06	7,30	3,68	4,56	3,89
Significance	1%		1%		1%	

Table 2. Relation red/green (a) at evaluated surfaces.

	Udder white		Teat white		Teat black	
	unclean	clean	unclean	clean	unclean	clean
n	23	23	34	34	19	19
Average	3,7	3,5	4,3	4,3	2,0	1,9
s	1,39	1,40	1,34	2,12	1,05	0,67
Significance	n.s.		n.s.		n.s.	

The parameter red/green (Table 2) generally produced positive figures, indicating a shift towards red. There was almost no variation due to cleaning.

The parameter yellow/blue did not behave in a uniform way due to cleaning (Table 3). All evaluated surfaces were dominated by yellow, indicated by positive figures. Cleaning white surfaces did not cause modifications of the parameter, but a significant reduction of the proportion of yellow was found after cleaning black teats.

Table 3. Relation yellow/blue (b) at evaluated surfaces.

	Udder white		Teat white		Teat black	
	unclean	clean	unclean	clean	unclean	clean
n	23	23	34	34	19	19
Average	14,6	14,6	13,6	14,3	7,5	3,1
s	3,30	3,31	4,04	2,84	3,16	1,29
Significance		n.s.		n.s.		n.s.

Corresponding to visual inspection by milkers the level of reflected light seemed to be best suited for evaluating the cleanliness of udder and teats. The numerical range of that parameter, found on teat surfaces, is presented in Figure 1. Clean white and black surfaces produced clearly different results. Results of unclean surfaces of both types were placed between the ranges found for clean surfaces. This structure of data is leading to the conclusion that non-linear procedures may be helpful to define the efficiency of cleaning activities. However, incorrect interpretation of data cannot be completely excluded.

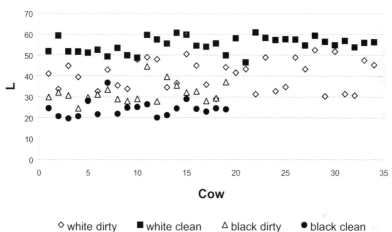

◇ white dirty ■ white clean △ black dirty ● black clean

Figure 1. Reflectivity (L) of evaluated teat surfaces.

Bloodstained surfaces

In tables 4 to 6 the results obtained at bloodstained surfaces are presented.
White surfaces of udder and teats before and after cleaning for all parameters produced significant differences of results.
As expected the parameter red/green was the most suitable one to detect contamination with blood. Furthermore it was the only parameter that was useful to evaluate the status of black teats with any certainty. When a level of 4 was exceeded then there was a high probability of blood being present on the surface evaluated (Figure 2).

Table 4. Reflectivity (L) of bloodstained surfaces.

	Udder white		Teat white		Teat black	
	unclean	clean	unclean	clean	unclean	clean
n	13	13	7	7	6	6
Average	36,3	62,0	45,0	57,4	19,8	22,8
s	5,29	4,10	4,14	2,48	3,98	3,41
Significance	1%		1%		n.s.	

Table 5. Relation red/green (a) of bloodstained surfaces.

	Udder white		Teat white		Teat black	
	unclean	clean	unclean	clean	unclean	clean
n	13	13	7	7	6	6
Average	29,5	4,4	13,9	3,0	6,3	2,3
s	6,11	2,36	2,28	1,68	3,79	0,71
Significance	1%		1%		5%	

Table 6. Relation yellow/blue (b) of bloodstained surfaces.

	Udder white		Teat white		Teat black	
	unclean	clean	unclean	clean	unclean	clean
n	13	13	7	7	6	6
Average	24,0	16,0	18,5	11,8	6,8	3,5
s	4,55	5,66	1,58	2,06	3,40	0,67
Significance	1%		1%		n.s.	

Summary

Evaluation of cleaning efficiency of udder and teats by spectroscopic parameters indicated an obvious change of intensity of reflected light after manual cleaning. The parameters red/green and yellow/blue were not useful to indicate cleaning efficiency at white surfaces. A significant reduction of the parameter yellow after cleaning was only observed at teats with black surfaces. Bloodstained surfaces were indicated by the parameter red/green in a most complete way. For this parameter an indication for a threshold value for bloodstained surfaces was found, independent from pigments at teats evaluated.

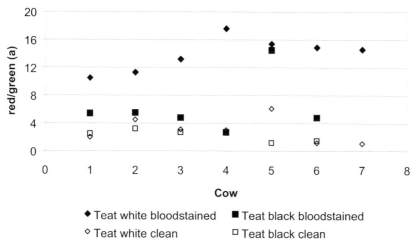

Figure 2. Relation red/green (a) of bloodstained surfaces.

Conclusions

The investigations described indicate, similar to results obtained by Bull et al. (1995) and by Bull et al. (1996), that spectroscopic parameters, defined in industrial standards, may be useful to evaluate the cleanliness of udders and teats and to detect the presence of blood.

The measuring device used for the basic investigations described in this paper requires mechanical contact with surfaces to be evaluated. It therefore is not suitable for automatic data recording under practical conditions.

Corresponding to statements of Bull et al. (1996) an image processing system, adapted to the inhomogeneous structure of surfaces of udder and teats, would be a more appropriate technical solution.

A more practical evaluation of visual cleanliness of critical areas can be expected by application of image processing systems, using various optical aspects for scoring structures of surfaces.

References

Bull, C., T. Mottram and H. Wheeler. 1995. Optical teat inspection for automatic milking systems. Computers and electronics in agriculture 12 (2) 121 - 130

Bull, C.R., N.J.B McFarlane, R. Zwiggelaar, C.J.Allen, T.T. Mottram. 1996. Inspection of teats by colour image analysis for automatic milking systems. Computers and electronics in agriculture 15 (1) 15-26

Haiger, A. 1966. Biometrische Methoden in der Tierproduktion. (Biometric methods in animal production) Österr. Agrarverlag, Wien, ISBN: 3-7040-0744-7

Mottram, T. 1997. Requirements for teat inspection and cleaning in automatic milking systems. Computers and electronics in agriculture 17 (1) 63 - 77

Ordolff, D. 2001. Einsatz von Farbmessungen zur Bewertung von Vorgemelken. (Evaluation of foremilk by spectroscopy) Proceedings Conference: Construction, Engineering and Environment in Livestock Farming 2001, edited by M. Krause, Institut für Agrartechnik der Universität Hohenheim, pp. 218 - 223

The $IDEF_0$ functional modelling method applied to autonomous precision feeding systems for dairy cows

J.C.A.M. Pompe[1], S.J.M. Wantia[1], C. Lokhorst[2] and A.H. Ipema[2]
[1]*Wageningen University, Farm Technology Group, Wageningen, The Netherlands*
[2]*IMAG, Wageningen, The Netherlands*
hanneke.pompe@wur.nl

Abstract

Precision feeding of roughage and concentrates for dairy-cows seems feasible with current technologies. However, the design of such systems requires selection of relevant components, and of their associated capacity and location. Many aspects affect these decisions, and a multitude of inter-relations exists between these aspects and the components of the feeding system. This paper describes the application of the $IDEF_0$ (**I**ntegration **DEF**inition) functional modelling method to elucidate these aspects and their inter-relations. It is combined with a morphological chart to find feasible configurations for (autonomous precision) feeding systems.

Keywords: Feeding systems, dairy-cows, design, $IDEF_0$, morphological charts.

Introduction

Electronic cow identification systems, automatic concentrate feeders, automatic milking systems (AMS) and the accompanying management software are accepted technologies for many dairy farmers. At the end of 2001, worldwide more than 1100 commercial farms milked their cows with one or more AMS's (Koning et al, 2002). The technologies provide the opportunity to optimise the milk production and the concentrate intake of individual dairy cows. Feeding roughage, however, is still a daily time consuming task for dairy farmers, which is not fully optimised. Site specific management provides the possibility to optimise the production of grassland, while technology such as balers offers the potential to collect and store the grass harvest in separate qualities (Lokhorst & Kasper, 1998). This technology, combined with knowledge concerning the feed demand of individual animals, offers chances to tune the roughage supply to individual (groups of) animals in the herd. In order to be practical, this would require application of autonomous vehicles and devices. In this way the feed intake of dairy cows could be optimised, feed costs and labour requirement could be reduced and the flexibility of the dairy farmer to plan his daily activities could be increased. Systems to automatically supply feedstuffs or to monitor the intake by cows are commercially available (Griffith Elder, 2003; WIC, 2003), but references for *autonomous precision* feeding systems of complete diets were only found for experimental purposes (Devir et al, 1996; Ichito, 1998; AgrarsystemsGmbH, 2003).

An autonomous precision feeding system (APFS) will not only consist of the device that dispenses the feed, but will also comprise equipment to unload the feedstuffs from their storage units, to transport them and to prepare the feed portions for the animal(s). Different choices are possible for such devices: for example feedstuffs could be transported with different types of conveyors, with an automatically guided vehicle, with a rail or cable system, with bucket elevators, etc. The devices must meet the requirements and restrictions set by the cows, by the law, by the farmer, by the layout of the farmstead, the finances, the environment, the food safety, etc. Examples for the restrictions set by the cows are the feeding requirements, which include aspects such as nutritional requirements, feeding behaviour, animal welfare, the feeding strategy (how are the nutritional needs of the cows met) and the feeding method (e.g. group or individual feeding). The combination of all devices together will determine the feasibility of autonomous precision feeding, as well as the labour requirement for the system, the costs, etc.

The introduction of AMS's has shown that not only the milking robot itself but also the logistics of the system - such as the location of the milking robot in the barn and the routing of the cows - need careful consideration. Halachmi (2000) developed a behaviour-based discrete simulation model, which enables a designer to optimise facility allocation for barns with robotic milking. This approach makes it possible to design an optimal robotic milking barn, which meets both economic and welfare needs.

Halachmi's example led to the original goal of the study presented in this paper: to develop a discrete simulation model of an APFS. Such a model would make it possible to evaluate the effect of various configurations - composed of various devices, with varying capacities and varying locations - on the technical and economic feasibility of an APFS.

A first step towards development of a discrete simulation model was the generation of different configurations for an APFS. Options for devices to unload, transport and prepare the feed portions were reviewed and a start was made to generate and critically examine combinations of these components. This revealed that generation of sensible configurations for an APFS required a thorough analysis of the many inter-relations between the different components, and of the multitude of requirements and restrictions set by aspects from various disciplines.

A study on integrated design for agriculture by Plaggenhoef (2002) revealed that the $IDEF_0$ (Integration **DEF**inition) functional modelling method is frequently utilised in industry for functional modelling. This standard method supports the analysis of a set of related activities or functions with the emphasis on the relationships between these activities or functions. It results in a hierarchical series of diagrams, text, and glossaries cross-referenced to each other. $IDEF_0$ models form an important communication tool when discussing the analysis of a system (NIST, 1993). Al-Ahmari & Ridgway (1999) developed an integrated modelling method where $IDEF_0$ formed a basis for the design of a discrete simulation.

The above led to the objectives of the study described in this paper. These were:
1. to elucidate the aspects that are related to precision feeding and feeding systems, and which influence the design of an APFS for dairy-cows;
2. to evaluate the applicability of the $IDEF_0$ functional modelling method for precision feeding systems;
3. to generate alternative configurations for an APFS.

This paper is based on the MSc thesis of Wantia (2001) who focused on the feeding process starting with the storage of feedstuffs and ending with the moment the cows receive the ration.

Methods and materials

In this study the $IDEF_0$ functional modelling method was applied to analyse the various functions and their inter-relations in a structured manner. This analysis was applied as the basis to generate configurations for an APFS.

$IDEF_0$ diagrams consist of boxes (three to six) with two to four arrows (see Figure 1a). The boxes represent functions, activities or processes. Each function can be detailed into a new diagram, called a child diagram. The arrows represent data and objects influencing and inter-relating those functions (see Figure 1b). In addition to Inputs and Outputs, $IDEF_0$ includes Controls and Mechanisms that influence a function.

Input: data or objects that are transformed by the function - e.g. an unfed cow.
Control: conditions required for the function to produce correct outputs - e.g. feeding requirements; animal welfare laws; available labour.
Output: data or objects that result from the function - e.g. a fed cow.

Mechanism: means that support the execution of the function without being consumed themselves - e.g. a feed dispenser; a transportation device.

To indicate that objects or data influence two or more functions an arrow can be forked into two or more arrows.

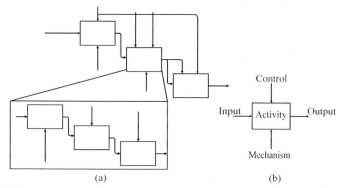

Figure 1. IDEF$_0$ Syntax.

Besides these diagrams, IDEF$_0$ models comprise glossaries, with a description of the terms utilised in the diagrams. These glossaries play an important role in the correct understanding of the model and support discussions with experts from various domains.

A literature review on feeding and feeding systems for dairy cows by Wantia (2001) formed the basis for our IDEF$_0$ feeding system model. Microsoft-Visio 2000 was used as a tool to develop it. A list was made of the options to realise the various mechanisms. The sub-functions from the IDEF$_0$ feeding system model and the options for their mechanisms were placed in a morphological chart (Cross, 2000) to identify possible configurations for an APFS. In the morphological chart different options were connected to find feasible solutions. The control arrows in the IDEF$_0$ feeding model served as a guide to check whether the solutions met the constraints and restrictions for an APFS. The approach to find new work methods by investigating the possibilities to *eliminate* or *combine* sub-functions or mechanisms, or *change the sequence* or *simplify* the sub-functions (Witney, 1996) was also applied.

Results and discussion

The available space in this paper allows presentation of only a small part of our IDEF$_0$ feeding system model. Figure 2 shows the *Feed Cows* diagram with the five functions *Unload feedstuffs, Transport feedstuffs, Prepare feed portions, Transport feed portions* and *Dispense feed portions*. In the complete model each of the five functions was detailed down to the lowest possible level; Figure 2 contains only the first level of details for the function *Prepare feed portions*. The *Prepare feed portions* diagram comprises five functions: *Transfer feedstuffs to mixer, Mix feedstuffs, Transport mixed feedstuffs, Measure feedstuff mix into portions* and *Transport portions*.

The morphological chart in Table 1 is intended as an example for the approach to generate configurations for an APFS - only part of the complete chart is shown, a complete feeding system comprises more sub-functions and the lists of options for the mechanisms are incomplete. The zig-zag line that connects the options in dashed boxes, indicates one combination of sub-solutions for an APFS; other combinations are possible.

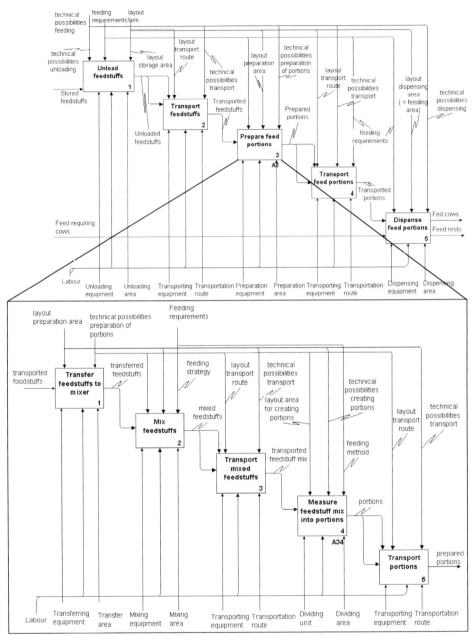

Figure 2. The IDEF₀ diagrams 'Feed cows' and 'Prepare feed portions'.

Table 1. Morphological chart for feeding systems with one possible combination of sub-solutions for an APFS, indicated with a zig-zag line.

Store feedstuffs	Unload feedstuffs	Transport feedstuffs	Temporarily store feedstuffs	Measure portions	Mix feedstuffs	Dispense feed portions
Horizontal silo	Scraping device	Tractor	Single-compartment hopper	Volumetric	Mobile unit	Along feeding fence
Vertical silo	Bottom unloader	Conveyor belt	Multiple compartment hopper	Gravimetric	Stationary unit	Responder station
Bales	Top unloader	Unit on rails		.....		station
Sacks / bags	Front loader	Cable way	Feeding lane		.....	....
Grass in field	Gravity	AGV	.....			
.....	Cow	Auger				
	.....	Pump				
		Air				
		.....				

An assumption that underlies this APFS configuration is the possibility to create individual rations by varying the fractions of feedstuffs - e.g. 50% grass silage, 40% maize silage and 10% concentrate, or 40% grass silage, 60% maize silage and 0% concentrate. In this configuration all the feedstuffs are temporarily stored in separate compartments in a hopper. When a cow enters the responder station, a gravimetric device measures the components that form her portion; the components are mixed and supplied on a "feeding tray" which is attached to the hopper. In this solution the mechanisms for *Store temporarily, Measure portions, Mix Feedstuffs* and *Dispense feed portions* are combined with the responder station.

When discussing this configuration with experts, they indicated that cows prefer to eat their feedstuffs in bouts and like to roam around while gathering their food. This behaviour implies that the separate portions should be small and that a cow should preferably have the option to eat at more than one station. This knowledge can easily be incorporated in the $IDEF_0$ model by further detailing the control "Feeding requirements" for *Dispense feed portions*. Such additional knowledge may affect the feasible options in the morphological chart; the options for the sub-functions that have "Feeding requirements" as a control should be checked. This demonstrates a strong point of applying $IDEF_0$: its graphical representation is easy to understand and stimulates discussions with experts from various disciplines. It is relatively simple to evaluate the effect of new developments - such as technological, social, legal - in an $IDEF_0$ model by adding them as new controls, or by detailing existing controls. Discussions with experts from different disciplines - such as animal nutrition, animal behaviour, environmental sciences, safety, etc. - are expected to make the $IDEF_0$ feeding system model more complete. In combination with a morphological chart, this can lead to new configurations for (autonomous) (precision) feeding systems.

The straightforward syntax of the $IDEF_0$ method is not difficult to master. The semantics however, require a thorough understanding of the method and the model.

Conclusions

The $IDEF_0$ functional modelling method can provide the necessary insight in relations between functions and related aspects that influence the design of an APFS. The combination with a morphological diagram makes it a valuable approach for generating alternative configurations for feeding systems, including autonomous precision feeding systems. This approach can promote communication and understanding between experts from different disciplines. New developments can easily be incorporated and evaluated.

References

Agrarsystem GmbH. 2003. www.agrar-system.de. 06-01-2003.

Al-Ahmari, A.M.A. and Ridgway, K. 1999. An integrated modelling method to support manufacturing systems analysis and design. Computers in Industry 38(3), pp. 225-238.

Cross, N. 2000. Engineering design methods: strategies for product design. Wiley, Chichester, 212 pp.

Devir, S., Hogeveen, H., Hogewerf, P.H., Ipema, A.H., Ketelaar-De Lauwere, C.C., Rossing, W., Smits, A.C. and Stefanowaska, J. 1996. Design and implementation of a system for automatic milking and feeding. Canadian Agricultural Engineering 38(2), pp. 107-113.

Griffith Elder. 2003. www.griffith-elder.com. 21-03-2003.

Halachmi, I. 2000. Designing the optimal robotic milking barn, part 2: behaviour based simulation. Journal of Agricultural Engineering Research 77(1) 67-79.

Ichito, K. 1998. TMR Preparation and automated feeding system in Japan. In: Proceedings of the Dutch-Japanese Workshop on Precision Dairy Farming, edited by C.E. van 't Klooster and K. Amaha, IMAG-DLO, Wageningen, NL, pp. 127-130.

Koning, K. de, Vorst, Y. van der, and Meijering, A. 2002. Automatic milking experience and development in Europe. In: Proceedings of The First North American Conference on Robotic Milking. March 20-22, 2002, Toronto, Canada, edited by J. McLean, M. Sinclair and B. West, Wageningen Pers, Wageningen, Netherlands. pp.I1-I11.

Lokhorst, C. and Kasper, G.J. 1998. Site specific grassland management: measuring techniques, spatial - and temporal variation in grass yields. VDI-Berichte 1449, pp 209-214.

NIST, National Institute for Standards and Technology. 1993. Announcing the Standard for Integration Definition for Function Modeling (IDEF0). Federal Information Processing Standards Publication 183. Www.idef.com/Downloads/pdf/idef0.pfd. 30-12-2002. 116 pp. Draft.

Plaggenhoef, W. van. 2002. Geïntegreerd Bedrijfskundig Ontwerpen; Utopie of Noodzaak? "Integrated Operations Design: Utopia or Necessity?" MSc Thesis, Wageningen University, Wageningen, The Netherlands, 148 pp.

Wantia, S.J.M. 2001. Developing a feeding system for dairy-cows; a methodological approach. MSc Thesis Wageningen University, Wageningen, The Netherlands, 90 pp.

WIC. 2003. www.wicideal.com. 21-03-2003

Witney, B. 1996. Choosing & Using Farm Machines. Land Technology Ltd., Edinburgh, UK, 412 pp.

Telemetric measurement and monitoring of animal welfare parameters and its importance for precision livestock farming

K.M. Scheibe[1], A. Berger[1], W.J. Streich[1], J. Langbein[2] and K. Eichhorn[1]
[1]Institute for Zoo Biology and Wildlife Research, PB 601103, D-10252 Berlin, Germany
[2]Research Institute for the Biology of Farm Animals, Wilhelm-Stahl-Allee 2, D-18196 Dummerstorf, Germany
kscheibe@izw-berlin.de

Abstract

The storage telemetry system (ETHOSYS®) is able to record automatically different patterns of behaviour such as activity and grazing over complete years. Collars with sensors and electronic devices identify the different behaviours based on advanced analysis of sensor-emitted signals. The resulting time series are stored in the internal memory. These time series can be transmitted on command by radio to a PC. The data can be downloaded at intervals like days or weeks at distances of up to 200m. Chronobiological procedures have been developed for analysing the resulting time series for deviations of level and rhythmic structure. Different kinds of disturbance, transportation stress, introduction into a new herd, wounds, high parasite load, or social stress could be identified by these methods. It was also possible to determine the time of lambing in free ranging mouflon sheep.
The system is especially convenient for free grazing animals or animals in large groups as in loose housing systems.

Keywords: telemetry, stress, adaptation, disease, ultradian rhythm

Introduction

It is often supposed that keeping animals in natural groups on pasture or in loose housing systems prevents suffering and stress, but health control and surveillance of general state may be much more needed and more difficult in these conditions than in conventional rearing systems (Busato et al, 2000, Spycher et al, 2002). Daily inspections give only momentary impressions, individual variations can hardly be identified. This is also true for wild farming or keeping animals in reservations.

Implantable transponders have been developed for health control and monitoring extensively kept animals (Puers et al, 1995). But traditionally, animal keepers evaluate the state of their animals by brief observation of feeding and activity. Continuous automatic recording of such simple parameters as motor activity and grazing may improve such observations substantially (Scheibe, 1991). External devices for behaviour recording may be simpler, may transmit results over longer distances than implantable devices, and also may be able to deliver meaningful information. On the other hand, behaviour records are more difficult to interpret than for example body temperature and require specialized analytical procedures. The chronobiological approach is particularly convenient for the evaluation of processes like stress, disease and adaptation from behavioural records (Scheibe et al, 2002). On this background, a storage telemetry system for continuous behaviour recording was developed and chronobiological procedures developed and applied. Examples are demonstrated from different species and different, close to natural conditions to demonstrate the function and performance of the system.

Material and methods

Telemetry

The telemetry system ETHOSYS® consists of recording devices in form of collars (ETHOREC), a communication station (ETHOLINK), and software for a PC or laptop (IMF, 1993). The ETHOREC collars (weight 200g) contain two sensors, one for acceleration and the other for position tracking of the animal's head (up or down). Acceleration is detected by a piezoelectric element. The head position of the animal can be identified by means of a posture detector (Type CW 1300-1/PEWATRON). A microcontroller with memory (RAM) is used for interpretation and logic decisions about the signal patterns from the sensor unit and data storage. Grazing or feeding is defined as any movement with head down, and additionally (more restricted) as a series of movements of defined intervals with head down. General activity is defined as any movement independent of the head position, while walking may be defined as movement with head up. These decisions are taken every second (I/O sampling) and the corresponding seconds summed during fixed analysis intervals. At the end of an interval, the results are stored in different channels and the procedure restarts. In this manner, time series (maximal 4000 analysis intervals) are stored in the memory. Four different definitions for behaviour patterns can be programmed during production as well as the duration of the analysis interval to meet the needs of the user. In the investigations reported here, the general activity channel and the movement with head down channel were used. A collar contains two AA-Li/SOCl$_2$ type batteries, assuring a lifetime of at least one year. For downloading of data, a bi-directional data radio link is used . This link consists of a transceiver in the collar and a second transceiver at the ETHOLINK station. This station can work with a whip antenna or for longer communication distances with a yagi antenna. It is controlled by a PC via the RS 232 interface. 'With a 5 - element yagi antenna downloading is possible over distances up to 200m. After downloading of a data set, the memory is cleared for further entries. The software is used for selection of collars for downloading, organization of the transmission process, and data storage in files. The function of the system has been tested and validated by parallel observation (Scheibe et al, 1998).

Data processing

For visual inspection and macroscopic analysis, data are organized in daily data sets by means of a procedure (plot) and plots are displayed by ECXEL. They show the duration of behaviour during the analysis intervals coded in colours or grey in daily records which are displayed one beneath the other. Based on this data structure, deviation in daily levels or switching from daytime activity to nighttime activity can easily be identified. For microscopic analysis, a program (wifostat) has been developed. It subdivides the original data file in data sets of 5 to 10 days, and develops from these files the autocorrelation function from which the periodogram (power spectrum) will be computed. From the periodogram, significant periods are identified (Andel, 1984) and used to compute two criteria, the degree of functional couplings (DFC) and the harmonic part (HP).
The DFC is defined as

$$DFC = 100*SP(harm) / SP(total) . \tag{1}$$

SP(total) denotes the sum of all significant periodogram ordinates (i.e., the variance assigned to significant periods). SP(harm) denotes the sum of those periodogram ordinates which are significant and harmonic to the circadian period (period lengths of 24, 12, 8, 6, 4.8, 4, 3.43, 3, ... hours). DFC obviously describes that percentage of cyclic behaviour components in the sample (in terms of variance) which is synchronised with the circadian rhythm. The harmonic part is defined as

Hp= 100*SP(harm)/St   (2)

In this case, the harmonic rhythms are related to the total of power of the spectrum (ST). As St includes all components of a spectrum, the Hp expresses the relation of harmonic components to the noise level in the spectrum.

Examples

In the following, examples from records are given from Przewalski horses in a semireserve, from red deer in a deer farm, from free ranging mouflon, from sheep on pasture and from alpacas in a zoo. In all cases, individual time series were recorded and analysed.

Results and discussion

Przewalski horses in a semireserve

An overview of long-term organisation of activity (A) and feeding (B) is given in Figure 1 for Przewalski horses. This example gives a good impression of hierarchic functional order and dynamic interrelation among the different components of the biological rhythms. It consists of a changing daily level of the behaviours during the year (reduced activity level during wintertime), of a 24h-component, of components related to sunrise and sunset and of varying ultradian rhythms. The plot demonstrates general day-activity, but in summer, activity and grazing are displayed also in late evening and during nighttime. Variation in grazing is obvious during the year and differs moderately from the annual pattern of activity.

Time series were recorded from one Przewalski horse during its stay in the zoo, its transportation to the semireserve and its subsequent period in the semireserve.. DFCs were very high during the zoo period, drastically lower during the period of adaptation, and slowly recovered to mean values

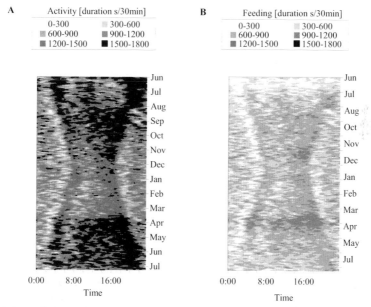

Figure 1. Annual plots of activity and feeding of a Przewalski horse in a semireserve.

which however were lower than the mean DFC of activity for the total herd during the same period of time (80.6%, Figure 2). Varying DFCs for activity, with a mean value of 85.5 %, were characteristic of Przewalski horse for up to two years from introduction to the semireserve. Somewhat higher DFCs occurred after two years (mean value of 90.3 %), and a more stable and harmonious activity pattern was visible. Starting from DFCs of 100 to 70%, a decrease to 40% and less at the beginning of June 1996 was calculated for all the individuals (four) recorded . At this time, a shooting yard was established nearby. The values recovered as noise insulation was improved.

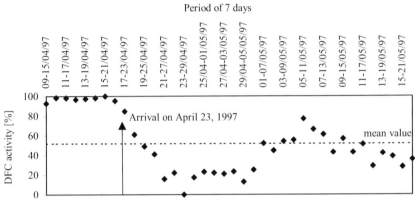

Figure 2. DFCs of Przewalski horse before and after transportation from zoo to the semireserve.

Red deer in a deer farm

Mean DFC values of a stag were 82 % for activity and 83 % for feeding (Figure 3). The DFC for activity dropped to 0 % on 21st August - the day on which the animal's antlers were cut off. The DFC for feeding dropped to 0% on 15th September and on 1st May - days on which the feeding regime was changed. A change of food led to minimum values of feeding DFCs but was of no impact on activity DFCs. This demonstrates, how disturbances can be detected within the functional behavioural circles affected by a specific external disturbance.

Mouflon in the wild

Lambing time in free ranging mouflon could be determined by an identification procedure, based on quantitative and pattern analysis of activity (Langbein et al. 1998). The DFCs from free-ranging mouflon normally were between 70 % and 100 % throughout the year. The lowest DFCs were always found in the week of parturition, a pattern which was found to differ with significance (p = 0.0006) from random distribution. At the same time, the activity level was significantly reduced (Figure 4).

Sheep on pasture

In sheep with parasitic infection, about one month before death structural changes could be found in activity and grazing. They consisted of reduced general activity and grazing especially during the night. In parallel, the noise - rhythm relation became gradually reduced as indicated by the HP, while the DFCs were reduced only during the transition period from high to low activity and grazing level (Figure 5).

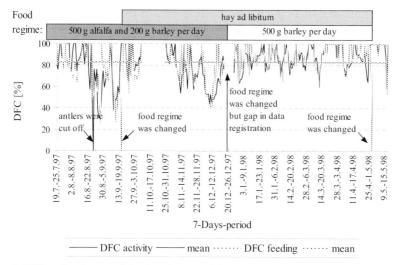

Figure 3. DFCs of activity and feeding from red deer in an enclosure.

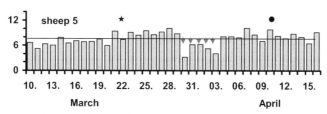

Figure 4. Daily activity budget of a mouflon sheep during lambing period. Asterisks indicate the lambing time.

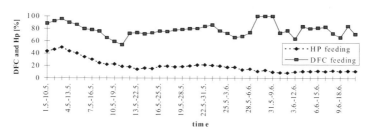

Figure 5. DFCs and HPs of sheep with parasitic infection.

Alpaca in a zoo

DFCs for activity normally were higher than 80%, while most values for feeding were equal or close to 100%. In an hurt animal, the DFC for activity was low as 28%, but for feeding stayed unchanged. The alpha female of the group was quite frequently engaged in social interactions and busy in care of all young animals of the group. Her DFCs at any time were somewhat lower than those of all other animals. Samples were taken from two females until just before parturition. DFCs were also lowered in these cases.

Conclusions

Stable rhythmic patterns have been described as basic precondition for animal welfare (Buchholz et al, 2001). All investigated animals showed a clear tendency towards a stable rhythmic pattern in normal and undisturbed conditions. DFCs and HPs can be regarded as a measure of internal and external synchronisation (Aschoff, 1969). They were found to be high in well adapted, healthy and undisturbed individuals but were lowered during periods of adaptation and by external disturbances or endogenous functional changes in all species and situations (Scheibe et al, 1999). The criterion allows for quantitative comparison between different situations, it can be used as a routine for scanning procedures.

The ETHOSYS system and the different analysis procedures can be effectively used in scientific research as well as in routine observation of high-value individuals or flocks under extensive rearing or wildlife conditions. The chronobiological approach is one way to compare and evaluate the quality of living conditions of animals quantitatively and to follow normal changes of general state such as birth or adaptation or annual rhythms. So it may become a useful tool for precision livestock farming.

References

Andel, J. 1984. Statistische Analyse von Zeitreihen (Statistical analysis of time series). Akademie-Verlag , 76 pp.

Aschoff, J. 1969: Desynchronization and resynchronization of human circadian rhythms. Aerospace Med., 40 844-849.

Buchholz, C., Lambooij, E., Maisack, C., Martin, G., van Putten, G., Schmitz, S., Teuchert-Noodt, G. 2001. Ethologische und neurophysiologische Kriterien für Leiden unter besonderer Berücksichtigung des Hausschweins (Behavioural and neuropysiological criteria for suffering with special reference to pigs). Der Tierschutzbeauftragte 2/2001, 1-9

Busato, A., Trachsel, P., Schallibaum, M., Blum, J. W. 2000. Udder health and risk factors for subclinical mastitis in organic dairy farms in Switzerland. Preventive veterinary medicine 44 205-220.

IMF 1993. ETHOSYS®, Instrument arrangement for monitoring the behaviour of vertebrates in the open. System description. Frankfurt/O.

Langbein, J.; Scheibe, K.M.; Eichhorn, K. 1998. Investigation on periparturient behaviour in free-ranging mouflon sheep (Ovis orientalis musimon). J. Zool., Lond. 244 553-561.

Puers, R., Wouters, P., Lapadatu, D., De Cooman, M., Geers, R. 1995. A microprocessor based injectable telemetry system for animal monitoring. Biotelemetry XIII 284-291.

Scheibe, K.-M. 1991. Rechnergestützte Bioindikatioren - Verhaltensanalyse zur Statusdiagnose bei Nutz- und Zootieren. (Computerized behaviour analysis of state in domestic and zoo animals). Monatshefte für Veterinärmedizin 46 341-348.

Scheibe, K.M.; Berger, A.; Eichhorn, K.; Streich, W.J. 2002. Zeit und Rhythmen - Umweltfaktor und biologische Struktur (Time and rhythm - environmental factor and biologic structures). Aktuelle Arbeiten zur artgemäßen Tierhaltung 2001, KTBL - Schrift 407 64-75.

Scheibe, K.M.; Th. Schleusner, A. Berger, K. Eichhorn, J. Langbein, L. Dal Zotto, J. Streich 1998. ETHOSYS® - a new system for recording and analysis of behaviour of free ranging domestic animals and wildlife. Applied Animal Behaviour Science 55 195-211.

Scheibe, K.M.; Berger, A.; Langbein, J.; Streich, W.J.; Eichhorn, K. 1999. Comparative analysis of ultradian and circadian behavioral rhythms for diagnosis of biorhythmic state of animals. Biological Rhythm. Research 30 216-233.

Spycher B, Regula G, Wechsler B, Danuser J 2002: Health and welfare of dairy cows in different housing programs. Schweizer Archiv für Tierheilkunde 144 519-530.

Modelling the nutrient cycle on grassland dairy farms

J. Schellberg and I.F. Rademacher
University of Bonn, Institut für Pflanzenbau, Katzenburgweg 5, D 53115 Bonn, Germany
j.schellberg@uni-bonn.de

Abstract

The effort of analysing the N cycle on grassland dairy farms can be considerably reduced by introducing simulation models. Using the GRASFARM model, the grassland based milk production and related feed concentrate consumption and N import for a given production level was simulated on 35 farms. Results support previous experimental findings on the interactions between forage quality, forage conversion into milk as well as feed concentrate and related N input. Moreover, the model provides a precise basis of the internal N flow and enables systematic testing of scenarios with changing farm specifications.

Keywords: grassland, dairy farm, nutrient cycling, modelling

Introduction

Intensive milk production on grassland dairy farms requires considerable input of high quality feed throughout lactation. In this respect, energy concentration and protein content are the most determining factors. However, grassland forage cannot provide energy concentrations high enough to satisfy the demand of high-producing cows. Farmers tend to compensate insufficient forage quality for high milk yield and purchase feed concentrates from external sources, thus charging the farm N balance. Resulting N accumulation may affect the internal N cycle of the farm and may also cause N surplus and environmental pollution (Taube and Pötsch 2001). Consequently, the N cycle and N balance on grassland farms have been subject of numerous surveys and experiments, indicating strong relations between N input and surplus (e.g. Jarvis 1993, Jarvis et al.1996, Kühbauch and Anger, 1999).

Research has to focus on management effects (e.g. animal diet, grazing practise, level and N content of imported feed concentrates, farm area) potentially reducing the N surplus without causing a significant decrease of milk production and economic gain. However, to answer this question, time consuming and costly experimentation is required. Computer modelling can support research and lessen the experimental effort. Most existing nutrient flow models consider only arable land, some include grassland, but none considers grassland dairy farms exclusively (Dou et al. 1996, Harrigan et al. 1996, Johnsson et al. 1987, Kirchmann et al. 1988, Reuss and Innis 1977, Rotz et al. 1989, Thornley and Verberne 1990, Wu and McGechan 1998). We therefore developed a simulation model, with which N fluxes between farm compartments (grassland farm area, forages, animals, slurry container etc.) can be reproduced. It also allows sensitivity tests to prove relationships between N cycle and the above mentioned management parameters.

Material and methods

Model description

The GRASFARM model (<u>Gras</u>sland <u>F</u>arm Simulation for <u>a</u>pplied <u>R</u>esearch and <u>M</u>anagement) encloses four sub-routines, (i) intake of forage, energy and protein, (ii) milk production based on grassland forage and concentrates, (iii) intake of feed concentrate and (iv) nitrogen excretion, losses and balance calculation (Schellberg and Rademacher 2001). The model comprises about 150 compartments in total. It includes input parameters describing farm and animal characteristics (table 1). Each of them can be selected by the user and can be varied step-wise in repeated simulation runs to process sensitivity analysis. With this, one can study the theoretical effects of changes of farm characteristics and management on the nutrient cycle in a virtual grassland farm. The software allows also to activate external data files containing daily data of forage quality and milk yield instead of constant values.

Table 1. Input parameters of the GRASFARM model (variable = values were adapted to individual farms, numbers = values were kept constant for all farms).

parameter name	value	dimension
number cows	variable	[ ]
live weight	650	[kg cow^{-1}]
number cuttings (silage)	3	[l yr^{-1}]
number rotations (grazing)	6	[l yr^{-1}]
begin grazing	120	[julian date]
end grazing	305	[julian date]
grazing time per rotation	I	[d]
residues from pasture (relative)	0.2	[ ]
residues from silage (relative)	0.02	[ ]
energy concentration of forage	variable	[MJ NEL kg^{-1} DM]
energy concentration of feed concentrates	6.9	[MJ NEL kg^{-1} DM]
protein conc. of forage	variable	[g kg^{-1}]
protein conc. of feed concentrates	140	[g kg^{-1}]
N deposition	20	[kg N ha^{-1} y^{-1}]
N concentration milk	0.0056	[g N kg^{-1}]
N excreta relative to intake	0.8	[ ]
N loss slurry (relative)	0.3	[ ]
N loss pasture (relative)	0.5	[ ]
daily milk yield	variable	[kg cow^{-1} d^{-1}]
yield	variable	[kg ha^{-1}]

The N input into the virtual farm comprises purchased feed, atmospheric deposition and N_2 fixation of clover, the latter depending on the frequency of cutting and grazing. In this study, N losses relative to N excretion are assumed constant, as informations on factors determining N loss are not available in this case. The model strictly separates summer from winter feeding as to happen either exclusively on pastures or in the cow house. The yearly grazing period is also selectable, but daily grazing time is unlimited. Grassland dry matter yield and herbage allowance is assumed to satisfy maximum dry matter demand and intake of the dairy cows including losses. Model simulation runs are executed on a daily basis providing 365 values for all variables over one year. Resulting tables and graphs list and chart daily changes of the variables. The model was edited using Modelmaker Software, Cherwell Scientific Ltd., Oxford, UK.

Precision lifestock farming

Grassland farm survey

We conducted a survey on 92 grassland farms in 1998 (Schellberg and Schockemöhle, 2000) in the Bergisches Land, a mountainous grassland region west of Cologne. From this survey we selected 35 grassland farms; they all supplement the available forage with standardised commercial feed concentrates exclusively, which facilitates a precise determination of the related annual N input. For each of the 35 farms a simulation run was conducted, using individual farm parameters as variable input (Tab. 1). Further, the amount of supplement concentrate consumption presumed in the model was adjusted to the measured consumption registered by the farmers. Thereafter, the energy concentration of the grassland forage was calculated from the residual energy demand for a given milk yield of the dairy herd. Additionally, an optimisation routine was run to adjust estimates of the individual grassland area per farm to the actual size. Mineral N fertilisation has not been considered in this study.

Results and discussion

Some of the farm and N cycle characteristics obtained from the survey can be interpreted without model simulation runs. One of the most prominent relations in terms of N balance is between feed concentrate input and milk yield. Increasing concentrate feeding was associated with an increasing annual milk yield per cow (Figure 1). On average of all dairy herds, 1 [kg] of concentrates yielded more than 1.6 [kg] milk. However, the scatter of the plotted data in figure 1 indicates, that the conversion of feed concentrate into milk varied considerably. It has to be reminded already here, that the contribution of milk produced with grassland forage relative to the measured annual milk total varied considerably between farms (see below). A more detailed analysis of the data set is given in Schellberg and Schockemöhle (2000).

An advanced interpretation of the survey data was achieved by subsequent model simulations mainly considering the relation between N input, milk yield, farm area and N output. The simulations showed at first, that increasing feed concentrate input charged the N balance on an area basis (Figure 2). The N surplus increased by about 0.03 [kg] per 1 [kg] input. It mainly derived from the accumulation of excreted N.

The offset of the regression line in figure 2 (b = 64.549) indicates, that the surplus theoretically never could reach zero, even if no concentrates and N would be imported. This contradicts with previous findings from balance sheet calculations based on similar farm data. However, in the present model simulations we reduced the percentage N losses on grassland to values expected with

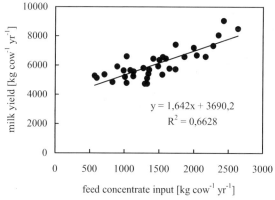

Figure 1. Feed concentrate input and related milk yield on 35 dairy farms in the Bergisches Land.

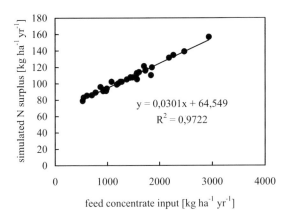

Figure 2. Simulated N surplus as a function of feed concentrate input. Each data point represents one farm simulation run.

the most advanced slurry application technique. As a consequence, the N balance values increased. Further, the mean N_2 fixation of clover on pastures and meadows was calculated about 40 [kg ha^{-1}], but neglected in earlier studies (Schellberg and Schockemöhle 2000). Naturally, any increase in farm area would raise the overall input of fixed N and N surplus in relation to the milk produced.

In figure 2, the scatter of the model data is low, indicating that the differences in N balance between farms, which use similar amounts of concentrates, is small. Consequently, there seems to be little scope to reduce the N surplus for a given amount of concentrate input. It is obvious, that any reduction in such input with the objective to reduce the N surplus would inevitably lower milk yield.

Taking up opportunities to improve the N cycle through management, an enhancement of forage energy concentration and conversion of self-produced forage into milk seems promising. We therefore studied the impact of forage energy concentrations on related conversion factors within the farms of the survey and found a strong dependency (Figure 3).

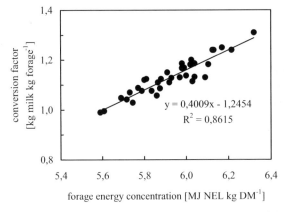

Figure 3. Simulated forage conversion factors for milk production of dairy herds as a function of offered forage energy concentration.

Precision lifestock farming

The GRASFARM model permits to calculate realistic conversion factors of forage into milk, regarding feed intake, displacement of forage by concentrates in the rumen and mean daily milk production. The farm survey provided a range of forage quality data wide enough to derive a strong relation between energy concentration and simulated conversion factors under the above mentioned actual on-farm conditions. Unless any influence of feeding technique and type of animal husbandary, farmers can expect, that the N surplus will be reduced with increasing quality of the available forage. In other words, the percentage contribution of grassland milk to the total obviously has an indirect effect on residual N from concentrates and on N balance (Figure 4).

Besides forage quality, the available farm area or stocking density seems an appropriate management tool to manipulate the N cycle. On per hectare basis, an increase in cow number improves the milk yield. However, it simultaneously increases the N flux from concentrate intake through excreta to the grassland sward. The extent to which such reflux loads the N balance,

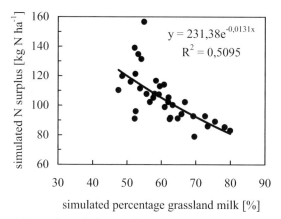

Figure 4. Simulated N surplus of 35 dairy farms as a function of grassland milk yield relative to the annual total.

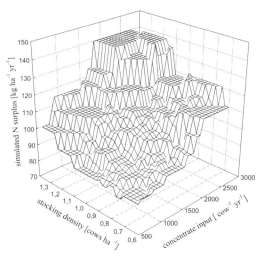

Figure 5. The effect of stocking density and feed concentrate input on N surplus of 35 grassland farms.

becomes clear from figure 5. Both factors, stocking rate and concentrate input, seem to have a similar impact on N surplus, at least within the sample and factor range of the survey.

Conclusions

A precise handling of nutrients in grassland dairy farms is a prerequisite of environmentally friendly production. The required precision on which farmers can count, depends on the available tools. Grassland models, often critised as being unrealistic or academic tools only, can provide priceless and helpful information, with which farmers may calculate their nutrient budget accurately. The GRASFARM model also provides an insight into the internal N cycle, thus far not presented.

Uncertainty of the model results mainly derive from the fact, that the necessary information about site-related factors are scarce. However, the most arguable farm information on grassland is still on dry matter yield altough it is - from the modelling point of view - a core parameter related with fertiliser demand, available forage, farm area and many others. Further, realtime decisions on nutrient input and handling requires not only informations on yield but on quality too. Therefore, we understand our model activities in context with online data acquisition, not yet available on grassland.

References

Dou, Z., Kohn R.A., Ferguson, J.D., Boston, R.C. and Newbold, J.D. 1996. Managing nitrogen on dairy farms: an integrated approach I. Model description. Journal Dairy Science 79 2071-2080.

Harrigan, T. M., Bickert, W. G. and Rotz, C. A. 1996. Simulation of dairy manure management and cropping systems. Applied Engineering in Agriculture 12 (5) 563-574.

Jarvis, S.C. 1993. Nitrogen cycling and losses from dairy farms. Soil Use and Management 9 (3) 99-105.

Jarvis, S. C., Wilkins, R.J. and Pain, B.F. 1996. Opportunities for reducing the environmental impact of dairy farming managements: a systems approach. Grass and Forage Science 51 21-31.

Johnsson, H., Bergström, L., Jansson, P. E. and Paustia, K 1987. Simulated nitrogen dynamics and losses in a layered agricultural soil. Agriculture, Ecosystems and Environment 18 333-356.

Kirchmann, H., Torssell, B. and Roslon, E. 1988. A simple model for nitrogen balance calculations of temporary grassland-ruminant systems. Swedish Journal of Agricultural Research 18 3-8.

Kühbauch, W. and Anger, M. 1999. Model calculations of nutrient margin for grassland farms with milk production. Agribiological Research 52 (1) 77-84.

Reuss, J. O. and Innis, G. S. 1977. A grassland nitrogen flow simulation model. Ecology 58 379-388.

Rotz, C. A., Buckmaster, D. R., Mertens D. R. and Black, J. R. 1989. A dairy forage system model for evaluating alternatives in forage conservation. Journal of Dairy Science 72 3050-3063.

Schellberg, J. and Schockemöhle, F. J. 2000. Optimizing milk production on dairy farms based on permanent grassland. In: Grassland farming - Balancing environmental and economic demands. Grassland Science in Europe 5 302-304, edited by Søegaard, K., Ohlson, C., Sehested , J., Hutchings, N. J. and Kristensen, T.

Schellberg, J. and Rademacher I.F. 2001. The impact of management on nutrient cycling in organic grassland farms. In: Organic grassland farming. Grassland Farming in Europe 6 267-270, edited by Isselstein, J., Spatz G., and Hofmann, M.

Taube, F. and Pötsch, E. 2001. On-farm nutrient balance assessment to improve nutrient management on organic farms. In: Organic grassland farming. Grassland Farming in Europe 6 225 - 234. edited by: Isselstein J., Spatz G., and Hofmann M.

Thornley, N.M. and Verberne, E.L.J. 1990. A model of nitrogen flow in grassland. Plant Cell and Environment 12 863-886.

Wu, L. and McGechan, M. B. 1998. Simulation of biomass, carbon and nitrogen accumulation in grass to link with a soil dynamics model. Grass and Forage Science 53 233-249.

A neural network for the analysis and monitoring of stress calls of pigs

P.C. Schön, B. Puppe and G. Manteuffel
Forschungsinstitut für die Biologie landwirtschaftlicher Nutztiere, Forschungsbereich Verhaltensphysiologie, Wilhelm-Stahl-Allee 2, D-18196 Dummerstorf, Germany
schoen@fbn-dummerstorf.de

Abstract

In recent years sound analysis has become an increasingly important tool to interpret the behaviour, the health condition, and the well-being of animals. This applies especially to stress situations. The paper presents a procedure that can classify stress calls of domestic pigs. Using linear prediction coding (LPC) an extremely compact short time representation of the call, with a relatively low effort of calculation and a low number of features (LPC-coefficients) was attained. Classification of the LPC-vectors employed artificial neural networks, trained with the LPC-coefficients of pigs' stress calls, other non-stress calls, and noise. After training the network was able to classify stress vocalizations of pigs in practical farming environments.

Keywords: animal welfare, stress, vocalization, neuronal network, pig.

Introduction

Farm animals' housing conditions may produce stress and impairments of welfare if biological needs remain transiently or permanently unfulfilled. Vocalization may provide a useful tool for evaluating the emotional state of animals, such as stress, under captive and natural conditions (Jürgens, 1979, Schrader & Todt, 1998). In pigs, the stress vocalization is a rather sustained cry with high-frequency bands. The analysis and classification of pigs' screams may deliver the species' and the individual's phonetic characteristics that can be attributed to a particular stressor. If information on this interdependence is given it will be possible to judge the individual stress perception of an animal and, thus, its state of welfare or suffering.

Up to now, no methods of analysis existed for the recognition of arbitrary sounds, because general solutions for extraction and classification were virtually absent. False or too few features from the sound signal may result in inadequate classification and too many features can overload most computers, especially if real-time capability is required. Hence, differentiated, well-adapted procedures are required for nearly every classification task (Schön et al, 1999). Here, a system is presented for the recognition of stress screams of domestic pigs. It combines linear prediction coding (LPC) with an artificial neural network as similarly proposed for the detection of pigs' coughs (Moshou et al, 2001). The system can calculate and record in real time while neglecting other vocalizations and sounds (patent pending). The results are documented in a time-related plot and a protocol. The applicability of the procedure was tested with two examples under laboratory conditions and with a comparison of two feeding systems under real farming conditions.

Methods

Linear prediction coding (LPC) as a method for feature formation and data reduction

LPC generates data as a time series derived from a continuous signal. A sound sample $x(n)$ out of a series is taken together with a previous sample $x(n-1)$. A linear prediction of the actual sample is formed as a weighted sum of the past n samples. The difference (prediction error), e(n), between the two samples can be minimized by introducing $a_1...a_n$ as coefficients (LPC-coefficients). For the calculation of these n coefficients we used the autocorrelation method and the Levinson-Durbin-Recursion (Pham & Le Breton, 1991). The LPC-procedure is formally equivalent to the source-filter-model of the vocal tract (Fant, 1970). The LPC-coefficients correspond to the filter coefficients of the tract. Hence the model is sensitive to variations of the resonance frequencies of the tract and indirectly to the motor efforts which are required to obtain them. For the detection of pigs' stress screams 12 LPC-coefficients, equivalent to the first 6 resonance frequencies, have been found to be sufficient (Schön et al, 2001). The LPC-coefficients formed a LPC-vector. The LPC-vectors were analyzed for time windows every 100 ms.

Artificial neural networks

The classification of the calls was obtained with an artificial neural network (ANN). We obtained good results using a supervised 4-layer Perceptron type (Rosenblatt, 1962) and Self-Organizing Feature Maps (Kohonen, 1997) taking the LPC-coefficients as 12-dimensional input vectors. The advantage of the Perceptron is, that a faster classification (necessary for real-time processing) is possible. A Kohonen network delivers a very good visualization of the structure of the used data sets.

Animals and Recordings

The ANN was trained with stress calls of pigs (German Landrace) of various ages bred and housed in the pig unit at the Research Institute for the Biology of Farm Animals in Dummerstorf. The vocalizations were recorded in a noise-reduced chamber with a Sennheiser MKE 46 microphone and stored on a Sony DCT-790 DAT-Recorder (Schön et al, 1998). Stressors applied were immobilization of piglets by holding them upright at the thorax and keeping them above the floor; of growing pigs by forcing them on their backs, and of sows which were held with a nose snare. These procedures can not only reliably elicit stress vocalizations as indicators of high levels of excitement but are also paralleled by hormonal and neurophysiological reactions that indicate stress, such as increased cortisol, adrenaline, and noradrenaline levels (Kanitz et al, 1998, 1999, Otten et al, 2001, Tuchscherer et al, 2002).
The handlings of the animals were carried out with attention to not affect the vocal properties. The network was trained with the recorded screams against non-scream calls of pigs and noise (Figure 1).

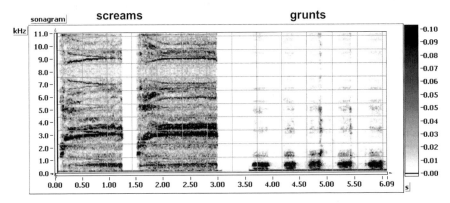

Figure 1. Examples of the used calls (screams and grunts) for the training of the network.

All procedures for data processing were developed and programmed using the graphical programming language LabVIEW® (Lab VIEW, 1998) with the additional tool Data Engine V.i.© (Data Engine V.i., 1999).

Examples for the applicability of the procedure

Example 1: Classification of individual piglets by their scream characteristics

The calls to be individually classified were recorded from 3 randomly selected piglets. They were housed together with their mother and kept in a standard farrowing crate. Stress screams were recorded on the fifth day after birth within an interval of two minutes per animal. This generated between 26 and 62 screams per animal for classification.

Training and test phase of the system: Fifteen screams of each individual were used to train a Self-Organizing Feature Map (SOFM) and a further 10 screams of each piglet were used to test the map. The maps used in this experiment consisted of 100×100 neurons and were trained in 3×500 learning steps.

The trained SOFM was then tested with vectors from screams that were not used for training. The results of the assignment of the test LPC-vectors is given in Table 1.

Table 1. Example 1: Results for testing the trained SOFM with unknown stress screams.

Piglet	No. of analysed LPC-vectors	Misclassification rate (%)
1	380	0.00
2	281	1.78
3	272	2.94

Example 2: Classification of piglet screams versus other calls and noise

First, stress screams of 19 piglets from 4 different litters (litters 1- 3: each with 3 two-week old piglets [training] and litter 4; 10 two-week old piglets [testing]) were recorded as described in Example 1. We further used the screams of 16 growing (five week old) pigs from two different litters (litter 5, with 9 five-week old piglets [training], and litter 6, with 9 five-week old piglets [testing]).

Second, grunts vocalized in various social situations were used (calls displayed in "non-stress" contexts). Grunts were recorded from 6 two-week old piglets (3 for training and 3 for testing) and from 6 five-week old growing pigs (3 for training and 3 for testing). Further, the nursing grunts of 10 lactating sows (5 for training and 5 for testing) were involved.

Third, two examples of the background noise occurring in the housing environment of the pigs were used. They consisted of arbitrary sounds (e.g. the talking of humans, air ventilation, and rattle of the equipment) without any animal calls (noise I for training, noise II for testing). All recordings were made randomly under normal keeping conditions in the experimental stable at the Research Institute for the Biology of Farm Animals in Dummerstorf. The recording equipment was the same as described in example 1.

The network was trained with LPC-vectors that were determined from screams of piglets and growing pigs. For the other class we used LPC-vectors from grunts of 3 piglets, 3 growing pigs, and 5 lactating sows, and noise I.

The SOFM used in this experiment consisted of 150 × 150 neurons and were trained in 3 × 500 learning steps.

The labelled SOFM was then tested with unknown LPC-vectors from screams (litter 4, litter 6), grunts (3 two-week old piglets, 3 five-week old piglets and 5 first lactating sows), and noise (noise II). The findings are shown in Table 2.

The results show that the classification of screams to the "stress area" occurred with a misclassification rate lower than 1 %. The grunts were to > 97.5 correctly attributed to the "non-stress area". A similar classification result was achieved with noise II.

Table 2. Example 2: Results for testing the trained SOFM with unknown calls or noise classified as "stress" or "non-stress" calls.

Animals (age)	n	Calls/noise	No. of analysed LPC-vectors	Type	Misclassification rate (%)
piglets (2-weeks)	10	Screams	1904	stress	0.58
growing pigs (5-weeks)	7	Screams	2476	stress	0.85
piglets (2-weeks)	3	Grunts	171	nonstress	2.34
growing pigs (5-weeks)	3	Grunts	245	nonstress	2.04
Sows (1st lactation)	5	nursing grunts	60	nonstress	1.67
Noise II	...	without animal calls	1706	nonstress	1.23

Example 3: Application of the system under real farming conditions

Subsequently the system was tested for its performance in a more realistic situation, applying it in a pig-plant in Mecklenburg-Vorpommern, Germany.

For this real-time application we used as a four layer Perceptron. Training of the network employed the same training data set as in example 2, supplemented by calls from sows which were held with a nose snare.

We compared the occurrence of stress screams in two different feeding regimes. In one case the animal-to-feeding-place ratio was 6:1 with 24 fattening pigs (average weight 50 kg) in a 4.85 x 3.90 m² concrete / slatted floor pen. This had a sensor-aided system where feed was added at a fixed time if the 1.50 m trough was emptied. In the second system enough feed was supplied once daily at an animal - to - feeding - place ratio of 1:1 (4 m trough) in a 4.0 x 1.80 m² slatted floor pen with 11 animals (average weight 80 kg). Stress vocalizations were recorded with a microphone (type: Sennheiser MKE 46) connected to a laptop. For measurement the microphone was placed 2 m above floor level in the centre of the pen and the system was allowed to record for two hours (before feeding, during the three feeding episodes and after feeding). In parallel a video system recorded the animals' behaviour and vocalization. In the resulting the Stress-Scream Monitor and Documentation Unit (STREMODO) records an increased screaming during the first two feeding sessions was detected with the 6:1 feeding place ratio (Figure 2a). The respective behavioural recordings displayed a high competition among the animals for the feed in these situations. In the third feeding episode the animals displayed less screaming and less competition, probably due to a more sated state. In contrast, in the stall with the 1:1 feeding place ratio the animals showed no detectable increase in screaming at feeding time as compared to other times when occasional fighting screams were detected (Figure 2b). These results demonstrate that the system is able to reveal the amount of stress vocalization in noisy stable environments and can be used for continuous monitoring of porcine stress calls.

The percentage of stress vocalization related to other recorded sounds was registered in 10 s bins, plotted on the screen and stored with date and time on a data file.

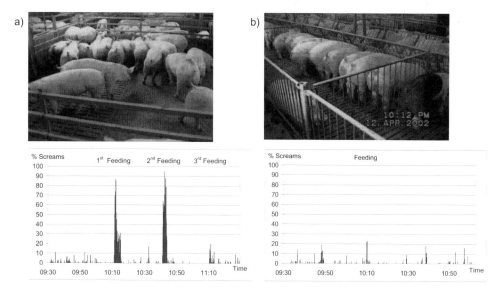

Figure 2. The temporal percentage of the duration of stress vocalization as recorded in the field test.
1) Restrictive feeding using a 6:1 relation of animals / feeding-place.
2) Trough-feeding with a 1:1 relation.

Discussion

The present procedure may be used as a methodological approach to solve different analysis and classification tasks in animal vocalization. It allows automatically monitored behavioural responses of farm animals in a housing situation with respect to their well-being or suffering (e.g. non-stressed vs. stressed). The procedure can be executed in pseudo real-time on commercial laptops. It is planned to develop a special stand-alone device that will allow continuous and objective measurement of the state of stress of farm animals, as long as it results in vocalization. In principle, the method is applicable for virtually all farm animal species that vocalize when stressed.

References

DataEngine V.i.© 1999. User manual, Function reference, Tutorials, Basics. MIT-Management Intelligenter Technologien GmbH: Aachen, Germany.

Fant, G. 1970. Acoustic Theory of Speech Production. Mouton: The Hague, The Netherlands.

Jürgens, U. 1979. Vocalization as an emotional indicator. A neuroethological study in the squirrel monkey. Behaviour 69 88-117.

Kanitz, E., Manteuffel, G. and Otten, W. 1998. Effects of weaning and restraint stress on glucocorticoid receptor binding capacity in limbic areas of domestic pigs. Brain Research 804 311-315.

Kanitz, E., Otten, W., Nürnberg, G. and Brüssow, K. P. 1999. Effects of age and maternal reactivity on the stress response of the pituitary-adrenocortical axis and the sympathetic nervous system in neonatal pigs. Animal Science 68 519-526.

Kohonen, T. 1997. Self-organizing maps. Springer series in information sciences, Vol. 30. Springer-Verlag: Berlin Heidelberg New York.

LabVIEW® 1998. Complete software documentation. National Instruments Corporation: Austin, Texas, USA.

Moshou, D., Chedad, A., van Hirtum, A., de Baerdemaeker, J., Berkmans, D. and Ramon, H. 2001. Neural recognition system for swine cough. Mathematics and Computers in Simulation 56 475-487.

Otten, W., Kanitz, E., Tuchscherer, M. and Nürnberg, G. 2001. Effects of prenatal restraint stress on hypothalamic-pituitary-adrenocortical and sympatho-adrenomedullary axis in neonatal pigs. Animal Science 73 279-287.

Pham, D. T. and Le Breton, A. 1991. Levinson-Durbin type algorithm for continuous-time autoregressive models and applications. Mathematics Control Signals Systems 4 69-79.

Rosenblatt, F. 1962. Principles of Neurodynamics: Perceptrons and the Theory of Brain Mechanisms. Spartan Books: Washington D.C., USA.

Schön, P. C., Puppe, B. and Manteuffel, G. 1998. A sound analysis system based on LabVIEW® applied to the analysis of suckling grunts of domestic pigs (Sus scrofa). Bioacoustics 9 119-133.

Schön, P. C., Puppe, B. and Manteuffel, G. 1999. Common features and individual differences in nurse grunting of domestic pigs (Sus scrofa): a multi-parametric analysis. Behaviour 136 49-66.

Schön, P. C., Puppe, B. and Manteuffel, G. 2001. Linear prediction coding analysis and self-organizing feature map as tools to classify stress calls of domestic pigs (Sus scrofa). Journal of the Acoustical Society of America 110 (3) 1425-1431.

Schrader, L. and Todt, D. 1998 Vocal quality is correlated with levels of stress hormones in domestic pigs. Ethology 104 859-876.

Tuchscherer, M., Kanitz, E., Otten, W. and Tuchscherer, A. 2002. Effects of prenatal stress on cellular and humoral immune responses in neonatal pigs. Veterinary Immunology and Immunopathology 86 175-203.

Comparison of grass sward dry matter yield assessment with imaging spectroscopy, disk plate meter and Cropscan

A.G.T. Schut[1], J.J.M.H. Ketelaars[1], M.M.W.B. Hendriks[1], J.G. Kornet[2] and C. Lokhorst[2]
[1]Plant Research International, P.O. Box 16, 6700 AA, Wageningen, The Netherlands
[2]Institute of Agricultural and Environmental Engineering P.O. Box 43, 6700 AA, Wageningen, The Netherlands
tom.schut@wur.nl

Abstract

The accuracy of an imaging spectroscopy system was compared with a disk plate meter and Cropscan (NDVI and WDVI) for non-destructive assessment of grass-sward dry matter (DM) yield. Experimental data varying in sward damage and N application were used. The disk plate meter resulted in R^2_{adj} values of 0.55-0.66 and Cropscan in R^2_{adj} values of 0.59-0.84 for NDVI and 0.47-0.65 for WDVI. Imaging spectroscopy calibrations resulted in R^2_{adj} values of 0.96-0.99, prediction errors (validation) were between 235-268 kg DM ha[-1]. Multiple observations may reduce errors strongly, with 27-68%. It is concluded that imaging spectroscopy performed better than the disk plate meter and Cropscan.

Keywords: Imaging spectroscopy, grassland, grass sward, reflectance, dry matter yield

Introduction

Currently, there are a number of non-destructive grass dry matter (DM) yield assessment methods available, such as rulers, the disk-plate meter (DPM), capacitance meter or crop reflection meters. The disk or rising plate meter is a thoroughly studied method for non-destructive DM yield assessment in grass swards (e.g. Gabriels & Van den Berg, 1993; Harmoney et al., 1997). Gabriels & Van den Berg (1993) concluded that the capacitance meter was not better than the DPM. The crop reflection, measured with Cropscan (Cropscan Inc.), is currently used for fertilisation recommendation in a variety of crops. The objective of this paper is to compare the accuracy of an experimental imaging spectroscopy system (Schut et al., 2002) with the disk plate meter and Cropscan for dry matter (DM) yield assessments in grass swards.

Materials and methods

Data of two experiments conducted in 2000 were used, where the degree of sward damage (experiment 1) and N application (experiment 2) varied. These experiments were conducted with mini-swards of *Lolium perenne* L., grown in containers of 0.9m long, 0.7m wide and 0.4m high, filled with a sandy soil (3% organic matter). The containers were placed under a rain shelter. Experiment 1 contained 36 mini-swards with 8 drought-damaged mini-swards, 12 artificially damaged mini-swards and 16 dense control swards. These sward varied considerable in ground cover- and tiller density heterogeneity. Mini swards were harvested by hand on 25 April, 12 May, 30 May, 20 June, 11 July, 8 August, 29 August, 27 September, and 31 October. In the N experiment N application varied in 5 levels, equivalent to 0, 30, 60, 90 and 120 kg N ha[-1]. This experiment consisted of two observation periods. Swards were harvested on 20 June, 29 August, 27 September, and 31 October. At harvest, fresh material was collected and weighted and dry matter content was determined by weighing.

In the experimental imaging spectroscopy system used, image-lines were recorded with three sensors measuring reflectance from 405-1650nm (Schut *et al.*, 2002). The sensors have a spectral resolution of 5-13nm and a spatial resolution at soil level of 0.28-1.45 mm². Schut *et al.* (2002) defined classes for soil, grass leaves (G), leaves with specular reflection (S), and dead material (D) and an intermediate class between soil and dead material. These classes are subdivided into reflection intensity classes (IC) with defined reflection intensities at 550nm, 800 or 1100nm (depending on sensor). After classification, spectra of pixels were normalised (Schut *et al.*, 2002), and mean sward reflection spectra were calculated per sensor. With this procedure only grass pixels were selected, eliminating pixels with soil and dead material. Ground cover was calculated per IC for pixels with grass (GCG_{0-6}) and grass with specular reflection (GCS_{0-2}) for each mini-sward. Total ground cover (GC, %) was calculated as sum of pixels in GCG_{0-6} and GCS_{0-2}, and was expressed as percentage of all pixels. The index of reflection intensity (IRI, %) was calculated as the percentage of GC that was classified as GCG_3, GCG_4, GCG_5 or GCG_6. A high value represents a dense canopy with more horizontally oriented leaves. The mean sward spectra and GC and IRI estimates were used for partial least squares (PLS) regression (Geladi & Kowalski, 1986). The data were divided into calibration and validation sets with a ratio of 2:1. PLS models were calibrated, and the models were evaluated with the root mean squared standard error of cross validation (RMSECV) and R^2 for calibration and root mean squared standard error of prediction (RMSEP) and Q^2 (comparable to R^2) for validation. The reduction in model prediction error ($RMSEP_M$) of imaging spectroscopy (S_{IS}) with multiple observations (N) was calculated according to:

$$S_{IS} = \sqrt{RMSEP_B^2 + \frac{RMSEP_M^2 + S_x^2}{N}} \tag{1}$$

The S_x^2 is the sampling error due to within-field variation. For an experimental field in the Netherlands this within-field standard deviation was estimated at 660 kg DM ha^{-1} (Lokhorst & Kasper, 1998). The S_{IS} was calculated with an intermediate (0.25) and high (0.5) estimate of the ratio between of $RMSEP_B$ / $RMSEP_M$ with 25 and 50 observations in the field. For this, the RMSEP averaged over the sward damage and N experiment experiments were used.

Sward height was measured with a plate meter at all harvests in both experiments. The rod was placed in the centre of the mini-swards and height of the foam plate was recorded. Both DM yield and crop heights were logarithmically (ln) transformed, according to Gabriels & Van den Berg (1993). At three harvests, on 20 June, 29 August and 31 October, crop reflection was recorded with a Cropscan (Cropscan inc.). The Cropscan records reflection in 8 bands, under a viewing angle of 28°. Crop reflection was recorded for all mini-swards in experiment 2 and for mini-swards with artificial and natural sward damage in experiment 1. The Cropscan was held 80 cm above soil surface, resulting in a field of view with 0.2 m radius. Means of two measurements, directed to opposite sides of the mini-sward, were calculated. The Cropscan was used in the rain shelter, what might have influenced the results slightly. The weighted difference vegetation index (WDVI) and normalised difference vegetation index (NDVI) are widely used for dry matter yield assessment. The NDVI was calculated as:

$$NDVI = \frac{R_{810} - R_{660}}{R_{810} + R_{660}} \tag{2}$$

where R_{810} and R_{660} is the crop reflection at 810 and 660 nm band. The NDVI is sensitive to optical properties of the soil background. The WDVI corrects for soil background and moisture content. The WDVI was calculated as:

$$WDVI = R_{810} - S * R_{560}$$ (3)

where S is the soil correction factor and R_{560} is the crop reflection in the 560nm band. For S, a value of 2.1 was used. Were appropriate, data were logarithmically transformed and an exponential or a linear relation was used for regression. The standard error of observation (SE) was calculated as the mean root square error (MRSE) of the residuals. For regressions on logarithmically converted data, the SE of observation was estimated with the relative error at the mean DM yield in the experiment.

Results

The variation in DM yield increased with crop height (Figure 1A). The sward height was linearly related to DM yield after transformation (Figure 1B). On log scale, the relative error was 32 and 39%, equivalent to an error of 555 and 645 kg DM ha⁻¹ at mean yields of 1733 and 1654 kg DM ha⁻¹ in experiment 1 and 2 respectively.The MRSE was 419 and 541 kg DM ha⁻¹ in experiment 1 and 2 (Table 1).

The mini-swards with high N supply in experiment 2 combined a high DM yield and sward heights below 20 cm due to lodging. The NDVI was exponentially related to DM yield (Figure 2A). The discriminating ability of this relation was severely limited above 2000 kg DM ha⁻¹ or 0.8 NDVI. The WDVI was linearly related to DM yield (Figure 2B). The variation in DM yield increased with WDVI value. Regressing a combination of all significant bands against DM yield improved results (Figure 3), with higher R^2_{adj} and SE of observation values (Table 1). Unfortunately, bands selected in experiment 1 differed from bands selected in experiment 2. The combination of GC and IRI had a strong linear relation (R^2_{adj}=0.82 and 0.89) with DM yield (Figure 4A, Table 1). Including also spectral information of leaves further strengthened relations with DM yield (RMSEP = 268 and 235 kg DM ha⁻¹ for exp. 1 and 2). Multiple observations within a field can even further reduce prediction error to 151-184 kg DM ha⁻¹ with 25 observations and to 116-158 with 50 observations in fields with a standard deviation of 660 kg DM ha⁻¹. In fields with a standard deviation of 300 kg DM ha⁻¹, errors were reduced to 95-142 kg DM ha⁻¹ (Table 2).

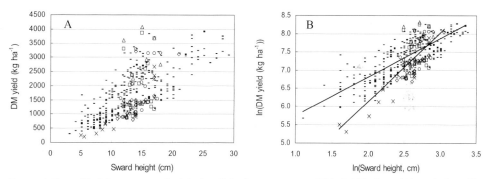

Figure 1. Sward height measured with the disk plate meter vs. DM yield before (A) and after (B) logarithmic transformation for experiment 1 (-) and experiment 2 for 0N (×), 30N (◊), 60N(○), 90N(□) and 120N(Δ).

Table 1. Regression equations for disk plate meter, Cropscan and the experimental imaging spectroscopy system for DM yield.

	Exp.	N #	Model	R^2_{adj}	SE
Disk plate meter					
Crop height	1	306	$e^{4.69+1.06\times\ln(\text{crop height})}$	0.66	555[*]
	2	98	$e^{2.35+1.90\times\ln(\text{crop height})}$	0.55	645[*]
Cropscan					
NDVI	1	44	$608+5.68 \times 580^{NDVI}$	0.84	163
	2	59	$248+2.41 \times 2687^{NDVI}$	0.59	689
WDVI	1	44	$420 + 41.5 \times WDVI$	0.47	298
	2	59	$70.2 \times WDVI$	0.65	638
Band combinations	1	44	$1208-117.0\times R_{460}+98.5\times R_{560}+25.3\times R_{610}-123.2\times R_{660}$	0.72	215
	2	59	$1567+328.7\times R_{460}-303\times R_{510}-199\times R_{710}+64.8\times R_{760}$	0.87	395
Imaging spectroscopy					
GC+IRI	1	334	$e^{5.19 + 0.028\times GC + 0.010\times IRI}$	0.82	323
	2	100	$13.94\times GC-174.9\times IRI+2.601\times GC\times IRI$	0.89	303
Spectra and GC+IRI[*]	1	147	PLS calibration	0.96	183
	2	37	PLS calibration	0.99	109
Spectra and GC+IRI[*]	1	73	PLS validation	0.93	268
	2	20	PLS validation	0.93	235

[*]SE approximated with RMSECV or RMSEP. For calibration R^2 values and for validation Q^2 values are depicted instead of R^2_{adj}.

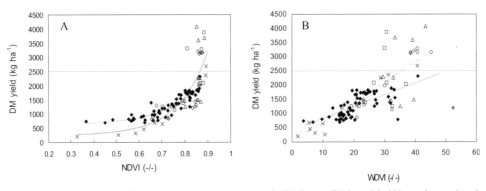

Figure 2. Normalized difference vegetation index (NDVI) vs. DM yield (A) and weighted difference vegetation index (WDVI) vs. DM yield (B) for experiment 1 (♦) and experiment 2 for 0N (×), 30N (◊), 60N(○), 90N(□) and 120N(Δ).

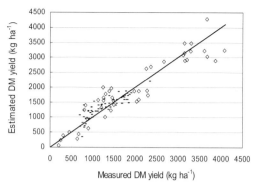

Figure 3. Regression result of combinations of Cropscan bands vs. DM yield for experiment 1 (◊) and experiment 2 (–).

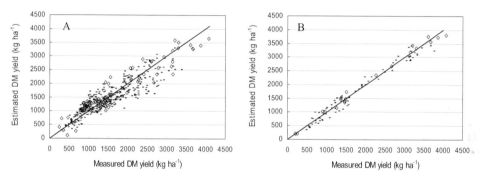

Figure 4. Measured DM yield vs. estimates of DM yield calculated with GC and IRI (A) and PLS calibration models including GC and IRI (B) for experiment 1 (◊) and experiment 2 (–).

Table 2 Potential RMSEP values at a DM yield standard deviation (SD) of 300 and 660 kg DM ha^{-1} for two ratios (R) between RMSEP$_B$ and RMSEP$_M$ and two observation frequencies (N).

R	N	300 kg DM SD (kg DM yield ha^{-1})	660 kg DM SD (kg DM yield ha^{-1})
0.25	25	95	151
0.25	50	80	116
0.50	25	142	184
0.50	50	134	158

Discussion

The standard errors for the disk plate meter were high. These errors were lower for Cropscan NDVI and WDVI in experiment 1, but higher in experiment 2 than for crop height. The large differences between the experiment 1 and 2 were due to different DM yield ranges, maximum yields were 2293 and 4075 kg DM ha^{-1} for exp. 1 and 2 respectively. The NDVI and WDVI were severely limited in their applicability at DM yields above 2000 kg DM ha^{-1}, or LAI 3-4 (King et al. 1986). Lokhorst & Kasper (1998) compared Cropscan with DPM for dry matter yield assessment in the higher DM yield range and found that the performance of Cropscan was not better than DPM. The required accuracy of DM yield predictions for fertilization and planning practices on the farm require a accuracy of 10% (mean deviation from the actual yield) (Sanderson et al., 2001; Lokhorst & Kasper, 2001). The prediction error found for DM assessment with imaging spectroscopy is promising for development of on-farm applications, especially when considering potential error reductions with replicate measurements (between 27-68%). These results are a significant improvement of other, currently available non-destructive methods. The number of sensors and the wavelength range required may be strongly limited when designing a system specifically for DM yield estimation. For practical purposes, extensive calibration and validation is required in order to account for differences in species composition and management practices, e.g. grazing.

Conclusions

It is concluded that the accuracy of DM yield assessment with an experimental imaging spectroscopy system was better than the disk plate meter or Cropscan. Imaging spectroscopy was less sensitive to lodging than the disk plate meter. Calibration and validations yielded strong linear relations throughout the DM yield range (300-4000 kg DM ha^{-1}), in contrast to Cropscan WDVI and NDVI estimates.

References

Gabriels P.C.J. and van den Berg J.V. 1993. Calibration of two techniques for estimating herbage mass. *Grass and Forage Science*, 48, 329-335

Geladi P. and Kowalski B.R. 1986. Partial least squares regression: a tutorial. *Analytica Chimica Acta*, 185, 1-17

Harmoney K.R., Moore K.J., George J.R., Brummer E.C. and Russell J.R. 1997. Determination of pasture biomass using four indirect methods. *Agronomy Journal*, 89, 665-672

King J., SIM E.M. and Barthram G.T. 1986. A comparison of spectral reflectance and sward surface height measurements to estimate herbage mass and leaf area index in continuously stocked ryegrass pastures. *Grass and Forage Science*, 41, 251-258

Lokhorst C. and Kasper G.J. (1998) Site specific grassland management: measuring techniques, spatial- and temporal variation in grass yields. *VDI Berichte*, 1449, 209-214

Sanderson M.A., Rotz C.A., Fultz S.W. and Rauburn E.B. 2001. Estimating forage mass with a commercial capacitance meter, rising plate meter, and pasture ruler. *Agronomy Journal*, 93, 1281-1286

Schut A.G.T. and Ketelaars J.J.M.H., Meuleman J., Kornet J.G. and Lokhorst C. 2002. Novel imaging spectroscopy for grass sward characterisation. *Biosystems Engineering*, 82, 131-141

Imaging spectroscopy for grassland management

A.G.T. Schut[1], J.J.M.H. Ketelaars[1] and C. Lokhorst[2]
[1]*Plant Research International, P.O. Box 16, 6700 AA, Wageningen, The Netherlands*
[2]*Institute of Agricultural and Environmental Engineering P.O. Box 43, 6700 AA, Wageningen, The Netherlands*
tom.schut@wur.nl

Abstract

The potential of an imaging spectroscopy system with high spatial (0.28-1.45 mm^2) and spectral (5-13 nm) resolution was explored as a tool for grassland management. Ground cover (GC) was strongly (R^2_{adj}=0.87-0.95) related to light interception. Growth and seasonal yield (R^2_{adj}=0.93) were monitored accurately. Seasonal means of spatial standard deviation of GC differentiated dense from damaged swards. Wavelet entropy of image line texture differentiated clover, grass and mixed swards. Drought stress was detected in an early stage and N deficiency was quantified with spectral parameters. Predictions of dry matter yield, nutritive value and nutrient contents (N, P, K) were accurate and robust. It was concluded that imaging spectroscopy can be a valuable information source for improvements of grassland management.

Keywords: Imaging spectroscopy, grass, white clover, stress detection, feeding value, heterogeneity.

Introduction

Farming systems under temperate climatic conditions mostly use grass as a major feed source and grassland management and productivity have a large impact on farm profits (Rougoor *et al.*, 1999; Vellinga & Van Loo, 1994). Currently, grass sward management on farms largely depends on qualitative expert knowledge. Information for management decisions (grass sward renewal or renovation, optimal harvest time, fertiliser application and irrigation) is derived from guidelines and rules of thumb. Reflection measurements provide information about various crop characteristics. Until recently, crop reflectance was measured at spatial resolutions much greater than the size of individual leaves. Imaging spectroscopy can provide detailed information on leaf reflection, ground cover, reflection intensity and spatial heterogeneity. Proximate imaging spectroscopy combines the potential of leaf reflectance, imaging and remote sensing as spatial resolution can be increased to sub-leaf level, severely reducing the effects of background on measured spectra of leaves (Schut *et al.*, 2002). Proximate imaging spectroscopy is very suitable for use within the framework of precision agriculture. It allows fast and automated data recording with mobile systems, providing means to quantify temporal and spatial variability at leaf-, plant-, site- and field scales. In order to interpret the meaning of variability, it is essential to know the relations between image parameters and agronomic variables.

The objective of this paper was to evaluate the potential of an experimental imaging spectroscopy system for grass sward characterisation. For this purpose, relations of image parameters with growth, dry matter (DM) yield, sward heterogeneity and growth capacity, white clover content, degree of N- and drought stress and nutritive value and nutrient content of grass swards were studied in various experiments with mini swards.

Materials and Methods

In the experimental imaging spectroscopy system used, image lines were recorded with three sensors measuring reflectance from 405-1650 nm at an height of 1.3 m above the soil surface (Schut *et al.*, 2002). An image line consisted of a row of up to 768 pixels and was at the soil surface 1.4 mm wide and 15.3 cm long. The sensors have a spectral resolution of 5-13 nm and a spatial resolution at soil level of 0.28-1.45 mm^2. In general, image lines were recorded two times per week during growth periods. Schut *et al.* (2002) defined classes for soil, grass leaves, leaves with specular reflection, and dead material and an intermediate class between soil and dead material. These classes are subdivided into reflection intensity classes. After classification, spectra of pixels were normalised (Schut *et al.*, 2002), and mean sward reflection spectra were calculated per sensor. With this procedure only grass pixels were selected, eliminating pixels with soil and dead material. Ground cover (GC, %) was calculated for each image line and mini sward. Reflection intensity varied with leaf angle and leaf height position in the canopy, as result of system design. The index of reflection intensity (IRI, %) was then calculated as fraction highly reflecting green pixels as percentage of GC. A high value represents a dense canopy with more horizontally oriented leaves. Spatial heterogeneity was characterised with the standard deviation over 42 image line GC estimates per mini sward (GC-SSD). The width of the chlorophyll absorption feature (CAW) around 680 nm of mean sward spectra was calculated as difference between half height of the edges near 580 and 710nm. Positions of minimum and maximum derivatives (λ_i) were calculated at various edges. Textural analysis was performed on reflection intensity values and quantified with wavelet entropy (Rosso *et al.*, 2001). Alternatively, a filter was constructed that separates continuous areas with green pixels between 10 and 25 pixels wide. The mean sward spectra and GC and IRI estimates were used for partial least squares regression (Geladi & Kowalski, 1986). The data of the sward damage and N experiment (see below) were divided into calibration and validation sets with a ratio of 2:1. Partial least squares models were calibrated and validation models were evaluated with the root mean squared standard error of prediction (RMSEP).

In 2000, experiments were conducted with mini swards of *Lolium perenne* L., grown in containers of 0.9 m long, 0.7 m wide and 0.4 m high, filled with a sandy soil (3% organic matter). In these experiments, the degree of sward damage, N application, water availability or clover content varied. The containers were placed under a rain shelter or in a climate chamber (drought experiment). The sward damage experiment contained 36 mini swards with 8 drought damaged mini swards (NDS), 12 artificially damaged (ADS) mini swards and 16 dense control swards (CS). Mini swards were harvested on 25 April, 12 May, 30 May, 20 June, 11 July, 8 August, 29 August, 27 September, and 31 October. The N experiment contained 15 mini swards and N application varied in 5 levels, equivalent to 0, 30, 60, 90 and 120 kg N ha^{-1}. This experiment consisted of two observation periods (1-19 June and from 8 August to 30 October). Swards were harvested on 20 June, 29 August, 27 September, and 31 October. In the white clover experiment, there were two mini swards with pure clover (*Trifolium Repens, cv. Blanca*), three with pure grass (*Lolium Perenne* L., Barenburg BG3 mixture), and four mixed swards. Two mixed swards contained more grass than clover (mixture 1) and two swards contained more clover than grass (mixture 2), but within both mixtures, grass was intermingled with clover. Swards were harvested on 29 August and 30 October. The drought experiment contained 9 mini swards and three treatments: control with high N supply (120 kg N ha^{-1}), and drought-stressed with high and low N (30 kg N ha^{-1}). Containers started with 20% (volume) soil moisture, where drought-stressed treatments received no additional water. Leaf DM content was measured for monitoring the degree of drought stress. At harvest, fresh material was collected and weighed and samples were taken. The samples of the drought damage and N experiment were analysed with standard procedures (weighing, near infrared spectroscopy and chemical analysis) at the Dutch Laboratory of Soil and Crop Research. Light interception (LI) was measured by hand with a Decagon LI-meter on clear and cloudy days. The tiller density coefficient of variation was determined with tiller counts in areas of 15 cm^2.

Results

Ground cover was strongly related to light interception (Figure 1). Including GC and IRI resulted in strong linear relations with R^2_{adj} of 0.92-0.95 for cloudy and 0.87-0.90 for clear sky conditions. Under cloudy sky conditions, intercepts and slopes significantly differed between dense and damaged swards, whereas under clear sky conditions, only the intercept was significantly different. Growth and growth stagnation were monitored with GC and IRI (Figure 2). GC showed a steep increase at low GC and smaller changes at high GC levels. IRI values typically increased in the second half of the growth period. Seasonal DM yield could be accurately estimated from regression with seasonal means of GC and IRI recorded just before harvest (SDM = 0.20×GC + 0.21×IRI R^2_{adj}=0.93, Figure 3). The tiller density coefficient of variation (TCV, tiller counts in areas of 15 cm^2) of dense swards (TCV=0.19 ± 0.02) was significantly lower than artificially damaged (TCV=0.52 ± 0.03) and drought damaged swards (TCV=0.74 ± 0.08). The TCV was related to the seasonal mean of the spatial standard deviation of GC (GC-SSD = 9.4 + 5.2×TCV, R^2_{adj}=0.69). The differences in heterogeneity resulted in significant differences in GC-SSD between damaged and dense swards (data not shown). The CAW parameter relates strongly to relative DM yield (R^2=0.95, Figure 4). The maximum derivative of drought stressed mini swards deviated from control swards before leaf dry matter content rose above 20% (Figure 5). The

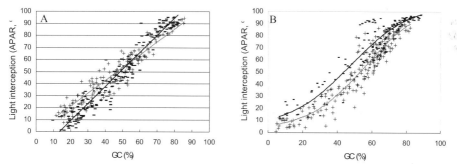

Figure 1. Ground cover (GC) versus light interception under cloudy (A) and clear (B) sky conditions for dense (-) and damaged swards (+).

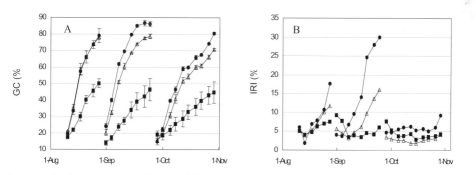

Figure 2. Evolution of ground cover (GC, A) and index of reflection intensity (IRI, B) for low (■), intermediate (Δ) and high (●) N applications levels.

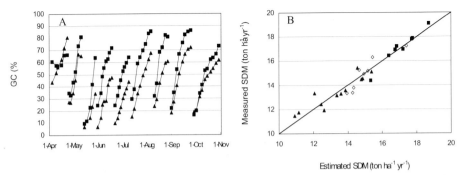

Figure 3. Evolution of ground cover (GC, A) for dense and artificially damaged swards and estimated vs. measured seasonal DM yield (SDM, B) for control swards (■), naturally damaged swards (◊), and artificially damaged swards (▲).

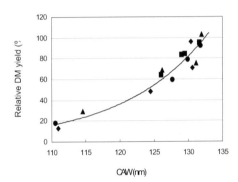

Figure 4. CAW vs. relative dry matter yield, symbols indicate harvests on 20 June (■), 29 August (▲), 27 September (♦) and 31 October (●).

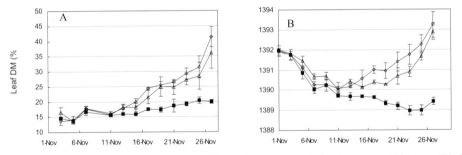

Figure 5. Evolution of leaf DM content (A) and minimum derivative near 1390 nm (B) for unstressed swards (■), drought stressed swards with low N (Δ) and high N supply (◊).

minimum derivative near 1390 nm decreased during unstressed growth, whereas edge movement of drought stressed swards reversed when leaves started to dry out. The wavelet entropy of image lines recorded in white clover swards clearly differed from image lines recorded in grass swards and mixed swards had intermediate values (Figure 6). With the filter, white clover leaves were

Precision lifestock farming

identified, but grass leaves perpendicular to the image line were also identified as white clover. The partial least squares model combining leaf spectra and GC and IRI estimates resulted in robust estimates of DM yield, DM content, crude fiber content and N, P and K content (Table 1).

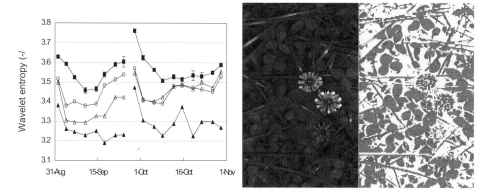

Figure 6. Evolution of wavelet entropy in grass (■), white clover (▲) and mixed swards (open symbols). The images illustrate classification result with the filter.

Table 1. Absolute error (RMSEP) and relative error to the mean (RE) for predictions of DM yield and contents of Ash, crude fiber, DM content (DMc), sugar, N, K and P for experiment 1 and 2.

	Experiment 1		Experiment 2	
	RMSEP	RE, %	RMSEP	RE, %
DM yield (kg ha^{-1})	268	15.3	235	14.4
Ash (g kg^{-1} DM)	6.5	7.5	5.8	6.0
Crude fiber (g kg^{-1} DM)	10.4	4.8	8.4	3.4
DMc (g kg^{-1} FM)	16.8	9.1	9.6	5.4
Sugar (g kg^{-1} DM)	16.2	13.6	27.7	18.7
N (g kg^{-1} DM)	2.4	6.2	3.4	11.7
K (g kg^{-1} DM)	6.0	22.7	5.1	14.5
P (g kg^{-1} DM)	0.50	13.2	0.62	14.8

Discussion

The recently developed imaging spectroscopy system (Schut *et al.*, 2002) provided valuable information about crop density, crop height, heterogeneity, image line texture and leaf reflection. In the moderate N supply range, leaf reflection is responsive to changes in N supply. Thus, differences between and within fields in N availability can be quantified with imaging spectroscopy, providing means for fine-tuning N supply to field-, site- or even spot-specific conditions. Drought stress was detected in an early stage. Spatial heterogeneity within mini swards was well quantified with imaging spectroscopy, providing means to characterise and monitor changes in sward quality. The successful separation of clover- and grass dominated swards allow quantification and monitoring of the fraction of white clover in mixed swards. Accurate assessments of feeding value and nutrient contents can be made. This opens up new means for improvement of grassland management and fine-tuning of rations for dairy cattle in the grazing season. It must be noted that the methodology requires further testing under field conditions, including a range of grass species and management practices before final conclusions can be drawn.

Conclusions

It is concluded that imaging spectroscopy was a valuable tool for monitoring and evaluating mini swards. It might also be a valuable tool for experimental and practical fields and may be an important information source for fine-tuning grassland management and precision agriculture on dairy farms. It provided means for quantification of standing biomass, seasonal yields, nitrogen and drought stress, sward heterogeneity, white clover content, feeding value and nutrient contents of grass swards.

References

Geladi P. and Kowalski B.R. 1986. Partial least squares regression: a tutorial. *Analytica Chimica Acta*, 185, 1-17

Rosso O.A., Blanco S., Yordanova J., Kolev V., Figliola A., Sschurmann M. and Basar E. 2001. Wavelet entropy: a new tool for analysis of short duration brain electrical signals. *Journal Of Neuroscience Methods*, 105, 65-75

Rougoor C.W., Vellinga T.V., Huirne R.B.M. and Kuipers A. 1999. Influence of grassland and feeding management on technical and economic results of dairy farms. *Netherlands Journal of Agricultural Science*, 47, 135-151

Schut A.G.T. and Ketelaars J.J.M.H., Meuleman J., Kornet J.G. and Lokhorst C. 2002. Novel imaging spectroscopy for grass sward characterisation. *Biosystems Engineering*, 82, 131-141

Vellinga T.V. and Van Loo E.N. 1994. Perspectieven van grassenveredeling voor bedrijfsinkomen en mineralenoverschotten [Perspectives of grass breeding on farm income and mineral surpluses]. PR-report 151, Lelystad, the Netherlands.

Sensor- supported cleaning and disinfection of the surface of

Automatic Milking Systems (AMS)

Jens Unrath and Otto Kaufmann
Humboldt- University of Berlin, Faculty of Agriculture and Horticulture, Institute of Animal Sciences, Division of Animal Husbandry and Technology, Philippstrasse 13, 10115 Berlin, Germany
jens.unrath@agrar.hu-berlin.de, otto.kaufmann@agrar.hu-berlin.de

Abstract

The use of Automatic Milking Systems (AMS) requires a change as well as progress in the management strategies of dairy farming. This applies in particular to the recognition of the contamination in relevant parts of such systems, because the farmer used to control the milking only in a random sampling way.

With the help of image processing it is possible to analyze changes in the degree of pollution of the surface. Relations between measurable contamination and the germ load can be analyzed. The investigation should be regarded as a first attempt to measure contamination of the external surface of the AMS.

This is important for the stabilization of the herd's health. Furthermore this should be seen as a step to a more consumer orientated production.

Keywords: Automatic milking, cleaning, disinfection, digital images

Introduction

One of the major goals of dairy farming is to produce milk under conditions characterized by a high level of hygiene. This level of hygiene is required by the milk industry as well as by the consumer. Since the mid 1990s AMS have become established in milk production. New management strategies are needed to run an AMS in an effective and economical way. Questions about the improvement of the hygiene management are of special interest. A number of research works are involved on the cleaning of the parts coming in contact with the milk but not for the external surface of the system. The higher frequentation of an AMS by the cows causes a higher contamination compared to conventional milking systems. This requires a manual cleaning of the AMS periphery several times a day. This is opposed to the expectations of the farmer, who wants to be independent of a fixed schedule. Therefore one often finds an AMS in a dirty condition between the cleaning times. This problem has to be solved, because it does not conform with hygienic production and the contamination represents a germ reservoir which can be dangerous for the herd.(PALLAS & WENDT 2001).

Digital photography and the associated image processing can be the basis for control of the cleaning and disinfection of an AMS. The work presented provides one approach to control the cleanness and the hygiene conditions by using image processing.

Materials and Methods

Our investigations took place on a commercial dairy farm with 115 dairy cows and two centrally placed AMS operating with free cow traffic.

The milking system Lely Astronaut has a mobile bionic arm. At this arm, shown in Figure 1, units for both cleaning the udder and for the application of teat cups are installed.

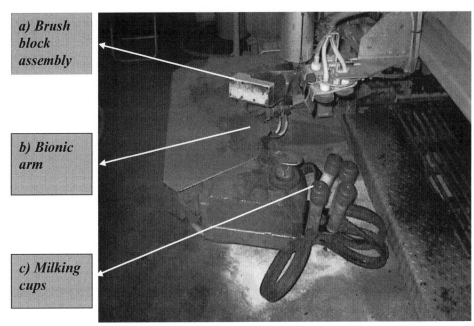

Figure 1. AMS in dirty condition, three relevant parts are shown :a, b ,c.

The brush block assembly as well as the milking cups are parts coming in contact with the udder and the teats of the cow (Figure 1 a,c). If these are obviously contaminated (including the bionic arm, Figure 1b), it can transfer pathogenic microbes to the entire herd. For this reason a), b) and c) are designated as sensitive parts and were selected for the test. Sources of the contamination of the AMS are skin particles, animal hair, fodder remainders, and liquid manure. They are carried mainly by the cows themselves into the system.

Digital pictures of these parts were taken (Hewlett Packard camera C 200, 1 million pixel, eight bit gradation of intensity) of the „Is- condition", the condition shortly after cleaning and disinfection (with Wofasteril E 400, 0.25% solution) as well as four and eight hours after cleaning (Figure 2). The term „Is- condition" describes the state of the system at the beginning of the investigation. That means the last cleaning dated back more than 12 hours.

The natural size of the digital pictures was 1152 x 872 pixels. The size of the examined details was 523 x 247 image elements. To ensure that the camera always viewed the object from the same angle, height and lighting it was used with a tripod and flashlight. The bionic arm was in its initial position. For the evaluation of the digitally taken pictures the program *Paint Shop Pro 7.04* was used. With the help of this program, difference pictures were produced.

At the same time swab- tests were taken to analyze the pollution on these parts of the milking unit.

Results

After more than eight hours of work without cleaning the sensitive parts of the AMS get considerably dirty. The load of bacilli, streptococcus, mould spores and E. coli. germs at the brush block assembly proven by swab-tests, lies for mould spores in a moderate and for all other germs in a high range. (Figure 2 at 11:25). The division of the y- axis in Figure 2 is based on statements of the Scientific Society of Milk Producer Consultants (MODEL, 2002.). It describes the success

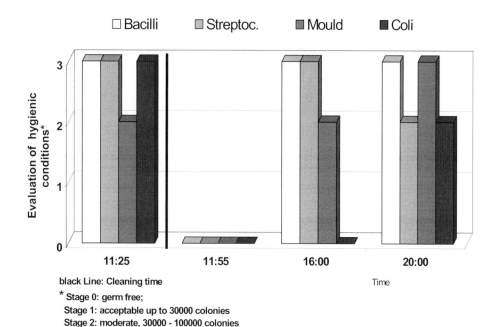

black Line: Cleaning time   Time

* Stage 0: germ free;
Stage 1: acceptable up to 30000 colonies
Stage 2: moderate, 30000 - 100000 colonies
Stage 3: unacceptable, more then 100000 colonies

Figure 2. Brush Block assembly: Development of the loads of Bacilli, streptocuccus, mould spores and E-coli germs in the course of time.

of the cleaning and disinfection of a milking parlour, by determination of the germ colonies after cleaning.

By cleaning and disinfection (with Wofasteril E 400, 0.25% solution) the germ load is reduced to a value almost zero (Figure 2 at 11:55). A renewed rise of the germs can be observed in the course of time after cleaning and disinfection (Figure 2 at 16:00 and 20:00).

This renewed rise of the contamination can be determined by the analysis of the digital pictures (Figure 3). Although analysis of digital pictures frequently requires the use of RGB channels (Red-

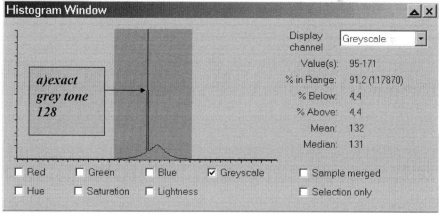

Figure 3. Histogram of the difference picture in the greyscale.

Green- Blue channel), in this application no significant difference between the use of color and the grey channel was found. Therefore the camera's grey channel was used.

The x-axis in Figure 3 covers the range from 0 (*black*) up to 255 (*white*) and the y-axis shows the absolute number of image elements belonging to the respective brightness value of the x-axis. The vertical line *a* in the marked rectangle represents the exact grey tone of 128 (middle of the x-axis). Four hours after the cleaning 91,2% of the image elements belong to a grey tone within the rectangle (Figure 3, % in range). This means that they are identical between both pictures. 8,8% of the image elements are not identical. They do not belong to any grey tone within the rectangle. (Figure 3, % below and above).

After eight hours, 9,6% of the image elements were not assigned to the value scale of the rectangle as seen in Figure 3. The both difference pictures according to four and eight hours after cleaning and disinfection show a modification of its image elements by 0,8%. This increase provides a measure of the rise of pollution of the brush block assembly.

As a conclusion from these values, it can be stated that the deviation of the image elements from the grey tone 128 is more largely, the more visible dirt is in the appropriate area.

Discussion

The use of image processing systems seems to be possible for the milk production with AMS. We found a clear relation between a visible contamination and the number of bacteria colonies on the surface.

For comparison of the pictures, it is necessary to take them at fixed points in absolute state of rest in order to keep all pixels congruent, because deviations in the pictures would lead to errors in the analysis and to wrong conclusions.

This is possible in an AMS by taking the pictures in the initial position of the bionic arm. A further possibility is to develop a robotic steering system for the digital camera connected with the frame of the AMS.

It has been shown that an analysis within the grey range is sufficient to represent the differences in the digital pictures (Figure 3).

However, the placing and the number of the cameras must be investigated. At present it is not certain that the selected points in the AMS are sufficient to evaluate the extent of the contamination. When a predetermined limit has been exceeded, either a signal must be given to the farmer to control the system, or a better solution would be to clean the unit automatically by nozzles near the relevant areas. It still has to be examined in which way these nozzles have to be installed and whether a possible warning system provides reliable data. The economic aspect of such a system needs to be investigated.

Conclusions

The use of AMS requires a management strategy for the recognition of contamination and an appropriate cleaning.

Although digital image analysis can register different degrees of pollution, it is still necessary to examine the extent to which this is sufficient to describe the degree of contamination of the entire system. This system can be considered as a possible tool, but it does not free the farmer from a duty to maintain the hygienic condition of the system.

Furthermore it has to be examined under which conditions the use of this system makes sense (e.g. conditions of light, number of cleaning nozzles, camera position, economic aspect).

Our investigation should be seen as a first step to an improved cleaning system of AMS. On the basis of these results, it is necessary to carry out further studies in order to be able to give more precise statements.

References

Hemming, J. 1998. Reihenerkennung im Pflanzenbau mit Hilfe der Computerbildanalyse. (Detecting the row structures in crop farming using image analysis) In: Computer- Bildanalyse in der Landwirtschaft. Workshop 1998. Bornimer Agrartechnische Berichte Heft 19, S.25-35

Hinz, A. 2000. Einsatz von automatischen Bildverarbeitungssystemen in der Fleischwirtschaft. (Use of automatic image processing systems in slaughtering industry) In: Computer- Bildanalyse in der Landwirtschaft. Workshop 1999/2000. Bornimer Agrartechnische Berichte Heft 25, S.68-72 Bornimer Agrartechnische Berichte Heft 25

Jähne, B. 1993. Digitale Bildverarbeitung (Digitale image processing), Springer Verlag

Model, I. 2002. Möglichkeiten zur Überprüfung und Auswertung von Hygienemaßnahmen im Melkbereich. (Possibilities for the examination and evaluation of hygiene measures in the milking palour) Tagungsband: Jahrestagung der Wissenschaftlichen Gesellschaft der Milcherzeugerberater e.V., 17.-18.09.02 Dresden, S.28-32

Pallas, S. and Wendt, K. 2001. The development of the udder health of a dairy cow herd in automatic milking systems. In: Physiological and technical aspects of machine milking. International conference, Nitra 26-27.06.2001. Proc 175-179

Secure identification, source verification of livestock - The value of retinal images and GPS

J.C. Whittier[1,2], J.A. Shadduck[1] and B.L. Golden[1,2]
[1]Optibrand Ltd., LLC, 1 Old Town Square, Suite 700, Fort Collins, CO 80524 USA
[2]Department of Animal Science, Colorado State University, Fort Collins, CO 80523 USA
jwhittier@optibrand.com

Abstract

Secure source verification of livestock is needed to assure food safety and high quality retail meat products; prevent fraud in animal subsidy programs; and enable effective source verification systems for control of animal diseases. A solution that will meet these diverse needs must; 1) resist fraud and include information on location as well as identity, 2) be based on a robust biometric marker, 3) allow rapid, economic and accurate acquisition of needed biometric information, 4) enable the data to be easily and rapidly transmitted, stored and retrieved, and 5) be humane and non-invasive. This paper describes use of digital images of retinal vascular patterns combined with Global Positioning Satellite systems (GPS) as a method that meets these criteria.

Keywords: Secure source verification of livestock, retinal imaging, livestock identification, GPS

Introduction

Source verification and identification of animals has long been a concern in the livestock industry. Recently, however, it has become an important global issue, attracting the attention of governments and regulatory agencies, food safety agencies, retailers and consumers. Widespread outbreaks and publicity surrounding bovine spongiform encephalopathy (BSE), foot and mouth disease (FMD) and swine fever have renewed interest in secure identity preservation and source verification methods for livestock. Verifying the source of livestock is important for food safety, continuous improvement in cooperative supply chain marketing programs, disease surveillance, fraud prevention in animal subsidy programs and country of origin labeling issues. Demand for secure identity preservations systems will continue as consumers, retailers, vertically integrated programs and governments expect dramatic improvements in all of these areas.

Identification (who is X?) and verification (is this X?) differ significantly (Woodward et al., 2001). The system described in this paper uses a biometric marker (the retinal vascular pattern (RVP) of livestock) to answer both of these questions as they pertain to livestock. Such a system must; 1) resist fraud and include information on location as well as identity, 2) be based on a robust biometric marker, 3) allow rapid, economic and accurate acquisition of needed biometric information, 4) enable the data to be easily and rapidly transmitted, stored and retrieved, and 5) be humane and non-invasive. Golden (1998) stated that only a biometric method of livestock ID will satisfy the requirements of producers to have a system that is not burdensome and of consumers who desire that the system be reliable.

Woodward et al. (2001) defined a biometric identifier as "any measurable, robust, distinctive physical characteristic...that can be used to identify the claimed identity of the individual". Practically, using a digital image of the retina is an economic, reliable method because the RVPs are unique, permanent, easily obtained and easily digitized.

This paper describes the development of a system by Optibrand Ltd, LLC, which uses the RVP of animals as a biometric marker and couples this image with information of animal location obtained from Global Positioning Satellite (GPS) technology, to satisfy the above criteria.

Available biomarkers for use in animal identification

Retinal vascular pattern

The retina of the eye of domestic livestock has a visible pattern of arteries and veins, termed the RVP. The pattern in domestic livestock was categorized by De Schaepdrijver et al. (1989): as 1) the presence of a large vascular network in the major portion of the light sensitive portion of the retina; 2) blood vessels extending from the optic disk to the neighborhood of the jagged margin between the light-sensitive and light insensitive portions of the retina; 3) large and small retinal vessels; with the large arterioles near 100 μm and large venules near 200 μm, making them readily visible.

The RVP satisfies the requirements of a biometric identifier outlined by Woodward et al. (2001) in the following ways:

1) Measurable - the characteristic can be easily presented to a sensor and converted into a quantifiable, digital format using a low cost and readily available digital camera. Indexes can be created resulting from a hashing function to allow for rapid one-to-many searching.

2) Robust - defined as a measure of the extent to which the characteristic is subject to significant changes over time. These changes can occur as a result of age, injury, illness, etc. A highly robust biometric does not change significantly over time. In humans, the peripheral retinal circulation develops during the last trimester of gestation (Hogan and Zimmerman, 1962) such that the visible or unmagnified RVP is set at birth. Though less well documented, the same development appears to occur in livestock. In healthy animals any changes that occur after birth are at the finer vessel or capillary level. In humans, there are a few diseases (e.g., diabetes, hypertension, and arthrosclerosis) that may cause retinal vascular changes. However, the incidence of these or similar diseases in livestock is miniscule and not of concern. Bracken fern toxicity has been reported to cause hemorrhagic activity in the retina of sheep (Tjatur Rasa et al., 1999) which may compromise the ability to collect viable images of sheep intoxicated with bracken fern substrates. In order to overcome the potential implications of loss of an eye in livestock, the approach used by Optibrand is to collect images of both eyes at the time of initial identification. Thereafter, either eye may be imaged as the positive link to the record of the animal. An animal that looses both eyes as a result of injury or disease would have minimal commercial value in the marketplace.

3) Distinctive - In humans, it has been documented that no two persons have the same retinal vasculature pattern (Simon and Goldstein, 1935). Additionally, Prince et al. (1960) state that the vascular pattern of the retina is very different from one species to another.

Nose prints and iris scanning.

Other non-invasive solutions of individual animal identification include nose prints and iris scanning. Technical challenges associated with collecting non-smudged nose prints from cattle have ruled out its use as an effective method of livestock identification (Biotech, 2000). Iris recognition technology has been developed for commercial use in humans and has been tested in animals. Granular imperfections at the periphery of the pupil provide unique differences to individual eyes. Use of iris recognition for animal identification is limited by the fact that the iris pattern does not stabilize until the animal is several months old and the iris can undergo alteration following injury or infection (Biotech 2002).

DNA profiling

This technique is already in use in pedigree animal breeding, particularly cattle, horses and dogs. Wider use of DNA technology in animal identification will be limited by the time taken to process samples (Marchant, 2002). Cunningham (2001) states that "until scanning the DNA of an individual animal in the field and generating a nearly instantaneous result becomes possible, DNA identification is unlikely to provide means of live animal identification." Additionally, Stanford et al. (2001) report a potential problem with the security of DNA fingerprinting as an identification method is that data may be falsified through improper sample attribution.

Other identification devices

Non-biometric devices that have been used in animal identification include injectable electronic transponders and electronic eartags. Since these devices are exogenous to the animal they have certain limitations compared with an internal biomarker.
Conill et al. (2002) evaluated the use of passive injectable transponders (PIT) in fattening lambs from birth to slaughter. Specifically they evaluated the effects of injection position, age and breed of animal. They reported that the injection of 32-mm PIT into the armpit or the retro-auricular region is not recommended as a practice for the electronic identification of fattening lambs, even though they perform similarly to small plastic ear tags. This is partly a consequence of the PIT losses observed on the farm but mainly because of the difficulties with recovering the PIT in the abattoir. Basarab et al. (1997) evaluated over 4000 yearling steers and heifers and reported a traceback success rate of only 39.8% from abattoir to feedlot and 46.4% from abattoir to herd of origin in a study using electronic identification (EID) eartags in Canada. The failure rate of the EID tags was low (0.12 to 0.21%) and dropout rates were measured to be zero in this study. The authors state that this level of reading accuracy and retention is adequate for practical application in the feedlot and on the farm. However, this study identified problems encountered in the abattoir that lead to traceback failure. These included hardware breakdown and incompatibility, software errors and incompatibility, plant logistics and electro-magnetic interference.

Materials and methods

The optibrand secure source verification system™

This technology consists of hardware and software that provide a *Secure Identity Preservation*™ system for livestock. The OptiReader™ device is a combination hand-held computer and ocular fundus digital video camera for collecting images of the RVP. The camera uses near infrared light to illuminate the ocular fundus and transmits full motion video at 15 frames per second to the hand-held computer. The operator sees the full motion video on the computer's LCD display.
The hand-held computer searches each frame looking for a single frame that it identifies as an acceptable image of the animal's RVP. When an acceptable frame is found it is presented to the operator for acceptance. The operator makes the final decision to accept or reject the image. The computer contains GPS satellite receiver board and antenna. The latitude and longitude, along with a satellite set time-date stamp, are encrypted and become part of the image record. This record also includes the device's CPU identification number. The device can be programmed to allow for additional user input of information (e.g. animal weight, sex, vaccinations given, etc.) that becomes part of the image record. The image and its accompanying data make up a data record called an "image blob" (binary large object). The image blobs are stored on a removable CompactFlash™ memory card. The OptiReader™ device cannot be initialized without an appropriately prepared card.

Global positioning satellite technology

The Optibrand™ system is use of GPS technology to mark each image with time, date, and location. This method allows individual animals to be identified unambiguously, with an extremely high degree of distinctiveness (Shadduck, 1999). Knowing, unmistakably, that a specific animal was at a specific location at a specific time is possible when retinal imaging is coupled with GPS. The Optibrand™ system uses this approach to establish a secure source verification process for implementation world-wide.

Data collection and analysis.

Digital images (n=625) of the RVP of cattle were taken with OptiReader™ devices. To obtain RVP images, cattle were worked through a squeeze chute in a normal processing manner. The user approached the animal's head and directed the camera into the eye. The RVP images and time to acquire each image for each user were recorded for later analysis.
A subset (n=52) of these RVP images were further evaluated. Branches from the left and right of the vascular trunk; total branches from the vascular trunk and total branching points showed differences across animals. In addition, a paired comparison of RVP from both eyes of 30 other animals confirmed that eyes from the same animal differ. Image acquisition data were analyzed using the PROC MIXED procedure of SAS with user as fixed and device and date as random effects. Least squares means and standard errors were computed accounting for unequal observations by user.

Results and discussion

Figure 1 depicts the RVP of a bovine collected with the OptiReader™. Note the distinct vertical trunk with branching vessels radiating from this trunk. Also note additional branching of the smaller vessels. The number and position of branches, along with the diameter of each vessel combine to offer an information rich biomarker for use in animal identification. Kinoshita and Honda (1991) reported that retinal angiogenesis is a Laplacian process which is ubiquitous in nature and follows branching patterns seen in rivers, trees, roots, and erosion channels.
Table 1 contains data describing the mean and variance of vessel branching in bovine retina imaged with the OptiReader™. Images from the subset of 52 random individuals illustrate the large amount

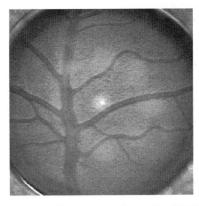

Figure 1. Digital image of the retinal vascular pattern of a bovine. This image depicts the branching and tortuous outline of the blood vessels that make each RVP distinct.

Table 1. Mean and variance of branching points in digital images of retinal vascular patterns from cattle.

	Mean	Variance
Random individuals (n=52 cattle)		
Left branches	6.4	2.2
Right branches	6.4	1.5
Total branches from the vascular trunk	12.8	4.3
Total branching points in the image	20.0	13.2
Paired eye images (n=30 cattle)		
Left branches	5.2	1.8
Right branches	5.2	1.8
Total branches from the vascular trunk	10.4	4.8
Total branching points in the image	16.5	14.3

of information available for uniquely identifying individuals using RVP. In addition, RVP images from both eyes of 30 animals were characterized and are shown in Table 1. Very large orders of combinations to distinguish animals reliably result from combining information about the relative positions of branch vessels, angles of branching and size of the branches. When number of branching points is coupled with position, diameter and proximity of vessel patterns, an almost infinite number of distinct information indices can be characterized.

Table 2 shows image acquisition data from six users using the OptiReader™. There was a significant ($P<0.05$) user effect in time to acquire images, the percent of images obtained in <25 and <15 sec. It does not appear that acquisition of images would add appreciably to the time required to process cattle. However, training and experience are important components for use of the OptiReader™ to successfully collect RVP images for animal identification.

Table 2. Least Squares Means of time required to acquire images by six different users using the OptiReader™.

User	n	Time to Acquire Image*, Sec		Images Acquired in <25 Sec*, %		Images Acquired in <15 Sec*, %	
		LSM	SE	LSM	SE	LSM	SE
1	81	41.7	6.1	56.3	7.5	35.5	8.8
2	40	24.7	8.8	71.2	10.0	58.0	10.7
3	279	25.8	3.9	67.7	5.0	42.8	5.8
4	169	27.9	4.4	69.2	5.5	50.7	6.5
5	10	64.6	15.0	24.2	15.7	7.1	17.1
6	46	93.9	7.9	28.2	9.1	20.1	10.8

*Significant effect of user ($P<0.05$).

Conclusions

The RVP of livestock is an information rich biomarker that meets the criteria of uniqueness outlined by Woodward et al., (2001). The process of obtaining RVP images appears to be compatible with other comparable livestock management practices. Using the RVP as part of a secure source verification process for livestock provide a humane, fraud-resistant tool for many applications in food production from livestock.

References

Basarab, J.A., D. Milligan and B.E. Thorlakson. 1997. Traceback success rate of an electronic feedlot to slaughter information system for beef cattle. Can. J. Anim. Sci. 77:525-528.

Biotech 2000. The Biotechnology Industry Annual Report, Burrill & Co.

Conill, C., G. Caja, R. Nehring, and O. Ribo. 2002. The use of passive injectable transponders in fattening lambs from birth to slaughter: Effects of injection position, age, and breed. J. Anim. Sci. 80:919-925.

Cunningham, E.P. 2001. Biological identification systems: genetic markers. Rev. Sci. Tech. Off. Int. Epiz. 20:491-499.

De Schaepdrijver, L., P. Simoens, H. Lauwers, J.P. De Geest. 1989. Retinal vascular patterns in domestic animals. Res. in Vet. Sci. 47:34-42.

Golden, B. 1998. Retinal Imaging: An un-alterable livestock biometric identification method. In: Proceedings, National Farm Animal Identification Symposium. Nov 8-10, 1998. St. Louis, MO.

Hogan, M.J. and L.E. Zimmerman. 1962. Retina. In: Ophthalmic Pathology, An Atlas and Textbook. Second Ed. W.B. Saunders. p. 475.

Kinoshita, M. and Y. Honda. 1991. The fractal property of retinal vascular pattern. Investigative Ophthalmology and Visual Science 32:1082.

Marchant, J. 2002. Secure Animal Identification and Source Verification. JM Communications, UK. Copyright Optibrand Ltd., LLC.

Prince, J.H., C.D. Diesem, I. Eglitis, G.L. Ruskell. 1960. Vascular System. In: Anatomy and Histology of the Eye and Optic in Domestic Animals. p. 57. Charles C. Thomas, Publisher, Springfield, IL.

Tjatur Rasa, F.S., T. Saito, and H. Satoh. 1999. The hemolytic activity of Bracken extracts in guinea pigs. J. Vet. Med. Sci. 61:129-133.

Shadduck, J.A. 1999. Animal Identification Technology Assessment. Unpublished document, June 1999.

Simon, C. and I. Goldstein. 1935. Eye disease and patterns of blood vessels of the eye. New York State Journal of Medicine. Sept. 15, 1936.

Stanford, K., J. Stitt, J.A. Kellar, T. McAllister. 2001. Tracebility in cattle and small ruminants in Canada. Rev. Sci. Tech. Off. Int. Epiz. 20:510-527.

Woodward, J.D., K.W. Webb, E.M. Newton, M. Bradley and D. Rubenson. 2001. Biometrics: A Technical Primer. In: Army Biometric Applications - Identifying and Addressing Sociocultural Concerns. Santa Monica: RAND. Appendix A: 67-86.

The importance of sampling time for online mastitis detection by using the electrical conductivity or measuring the Na$^+$ and Cl$^-$ content in milk

M. Wiedemann[1], D. Weiss[2], G. Wendl[1] and R.M. Bruckmaier[2]
[1]Bavarian State Research Center for Agriculture, 85354 Freising, Germany Institute of Agricultural Engineering, Farm Buildings and Environmental Technology
[2]Institute of Physiology, Technical University Munich, 85350 Freising, Germany

Abstract

Electrical conductivity (EC), Cl$^-$ and Na$^+$ concentration (Cl, Na) in quarter milk samples with and without clinical mastitis were investigated with two independent experiments. In experiment 1 milk samples were taken during pre-stimulation. In experiment 2 four quarters were sequentially sampled within 90 s according to attachment routine of automatic milking systems (AMS).
EC, Cl and Na in the first samples in experiment 1 were highly significant elevated (P<0.001) in high somatic cell count (SCC) quarters as compared to low SCC quarters. During the course of pre-stimulation differences in EC and CL disappeared or were restricted to significant differences for Na (p<0.05), due to the start of alveolar milk ejection. In experiment 2, the performance to detect an elevated SCC of more than 200.000 cells/ml was rather high in the first two sampled quarters, but was reduced with increasing time after the start of sampling. However, detection performance of elevated SCC can be improved by a combination of EC, Cl and Na measurements if the samples are taken within the first seconds after beginning the prestimulation.

Keywords: online mastitis detection, electrical conductivity, milk ejection, ionic content, automatic milking

Introduction

Electrical conductivity (EC) as an indicator for mastitis in bovine milk has been discussed for decades. The influences of the milking interval, milk fat or other constituents on the EC have been evaluated. Testing the first milk strips by handheld EC meters the sensitivity is between 70 and 100 % at a specificity of 95 % (Hillerton, 2000). However, without implication of additional parameters, e.g. the milk temperature, the performance of online EC measurement systems to detect mastitis was not satisfying (deMol & Woldt, 2001). Despite these shortcomings EC is currently the main parameter for detecting mastitis in automatic milking systems (Wendl & Schön, 2002).

In milk EC is mainly determined by the concentration of ions dissolved in milk, e.g. Cl and Na. Their concentration in normal milk from healthy glands is lower than those in blood (Schulz & Sydow, 1957). Minor effects are reported due to fat, protein and lactose as well as to the sampled milk fraction (Ontsouka et al. 2003). In the healthy mammary gland the mammary epithelial tight junctions are closed and the blood milk barrier is impermeable. In case of a mammary infection the tight junctions become leaky (Nguyen and Neville, 1998) to allow diapedesis of immunologically active cells to reach the site of infection. An inflammatory mastitis is associated with the damage of mammary tissue, resulting in a serious loss of integrity of the blood - milk barrier. Therefore, the content of Cl and Na as well as the EC increases. A threshold of 200.000 SCC cells/ml is defined to distinguish between healthy and disturbed secretion (Smith 1995).

The aim of this study was to test the hypothesis, that EC, Cl and Na in the milk of dairy cows is related to the sampling time relative to the first contact with the teats, i.e. the occurrence of the milk ejection. Additionally, EC, Cl and Na were analysed as a tool to detect elevated SCC in simulated AMS routines.

Materials and methods

In experiment 1 twenty cows with or without subclinical mastitis were investigated. Seven consecutive samples (~40 ml) were taken manually every 20 s during pre-stimulation (t=0 s first contact to the udder until t=120 s) in the right front quarter at three consecutive milkings. In experiment 2 quarter foremilk samples (~40 ml) of six cows were collected at 20 consecutive routine milkings in a parlour (milking interval 11 and 13 h).. The order of sampling was unchanged during the experiment to simulate the attachment routine of an AMS. Sampling started without previous teat cleaning at t=0s in right front quarter (RF), t=25 s in the right rear quarter (RR), t=50 s in left front quarter (LF) and t=70 s in left rear quarter (LR). Aliquots of the milk samples were analysed in the laboratory of the Milchprüfring Bayern e.V. for fat, protein, lactose and SCC (MilkoScan 4500, Foss Electric, Denmark). A volume of 2 ml of each sample for EC, Cl and Na measurements was stored at -20°C until analysis.

EC was measured by LDM 130 electrode (Wissenschaftlich-Technische-Werkstätten, D-82362 Weilheim) at a constant temperature of 25° C. Cl and Na were determined by ion selective electrodes (9811 and 9617BN, Orion Research, Beverly, MA USA) and were used in raw milk (Olmos et al., 1992; Randell et Linklater, 1972).

The milk samples were assigned to four groups according to their SCC in the first sample as follows: < 5.0 $\log_{10}$/ml *(SCC I)*, 5.0 to 5.3 $\log_{10}$/ml *(SCC II)*, 5.3 to 5.7 $\log_{10}$/ml *(SCC III)*, <5.7 $\log_{10}$/ml *(SCC IV)*. Groups *SCC II* and *SCC III* were clustered in experiment 1 to obtain an adequate number of samples in each SCC-class. Data are presented as means ± SEM. SCC was analysed as $\log_{10}$ to obtain normal distribution for further statistical analyses. Results were analysed using the repeated measures analysis of the MIXED procedure (SAS) and tested for significance (p<0.05) using the Least Significance-Difference Test (LSD).

In experiment 2, a sensitivity and specificity analysis was performed according to deMol & Woldt (2001). SCC detection target for sensitivity and specificity analyses was 200,000 cells/ml (5.3 $\log_{10}$/ml) to distinguish between healthy and disturbed milk secretion (Smith 1995). The individual quarter thresholds for EC, Cl and Na were set to reach a specificity of 90 %: i.e., no more than 10 of 100 observations with low SCC are falsely classified as "high SCC". *True positive* samples exceed the EC, Cl or Na threshold and had SCC of more than 200.000 cells/ml. *True negative* was defined as low SCC and low EC, Cl or Na. *False negative* was characterised as elevated SCC without exceeded EC, Cl or Na. Likewise, in *false positive* samples SCC was low while EC, Cl or Na were elevated. For combined evaluation of EC, Na and Cl an "or"-function was used for calculation of sensitivity and specificity.

Results and Discussion

In experiment 1 twenty-three quarters were assigned to *SCC I*, 14 to *SCC II+IIII* and 22 to *SCC IV*. Results are presented in figure 1. Average SCC in the first samples (t=0 s) were 4.62±0.07, 5.34±0.04 and 6.00±0.08 $\log^{10}$/ml in *SCC I*, *SCC II+III* and *SCC IV*, respectively. The SCC in *SCC IV* quarters was 2,520% (as absolute linear SCC) of the *SCC I* quarters before the start of stimulation (t=0 s). The SCC decreased throughout the measured period and was significantly lower in *SCC IV* and *SCC I* quarters 100 and 120 s after start of stimulation as compared to the start of sampling (t=0 s). The differences of SCC between *SCC IV*, *SCC II+III* and *SCC I* quarters throughout sampling remained significant at every sampling time.

The EC in *SCC IV* quarters was significantly higher compared to *SCC I* and *SCC II+III* for the first four sampling times (0 until 60 s). There was a clear decrease in EC between the 40 and 100 s after the start of pre-stimulation. The EC was significantly lower in SCC IV quarters later than 80 s compared to the start of pre-stimulation. The difference in EC between *SCC IV* and *SCC II+III* quarters disappeared at 80 s, whereas differences between *SCC IV* and *SCC I* milkings were still significant. In *SCC IV* quarters the EC was significantly reduced in samples later than 80 s compared to the start of pre-stimulation. Sampling later than 100 s after the start of stimulation resulted in similar values for *SCC IV*, *SCC II+III* and *SCC I* quarters. The EC before pre-stimulation (t=0 s) in *SCC IV* quarters was 121 % of the EC in *SCC I* quarters.

For Cl comparable proportions could be observed. The decrease in Cl took place between 60 and 100 s. At the start of sampling Cl was higher in *SCC IV* quarters compared to *SCC I* quarters, *SCC I* and *SCC II+III* quarters did not differ. Cl was similar in *SCC IV*, *SCC II+III* and *SCC I* quarters sampled later than 80 s. In *SCC IV* quarters Cl was significantly reduced later than 80 s compared to the start of pre-stimulation (t=0 s). Prior to the start of pre-stimulation in *SCC IV* quarters Cl was 141% of the *SCC I* quarters.

Na was significantly higher in *SCC IV* quarters compared to *SCC I* throughout the sampling period. *SCC I* and *SCC II+III* were similar for all time points. However as for the EC and Cl a dramatic decrease of Na in *SCC IV* quarters was observed. Na in *SCC IV* quarters was significantly reduced in samples later than 80 s as compared to the start of pre-stimulation. Na before the start of pre-stimulation in *SCC IV* quarters was 283 % of the *SCC I* quarters.

For all observed parameters (SCC, EC, Cl and Na) the values decreased dramatically throughout the time series of sampling. The values were constant until the third sampling (t=40 s), further they dropped down and reached their minimum after 100 s. Since the samples were taken during pre-stimulation it is obvious, that the start of milk ejection - the shift of alveolar milk into the cisternal cavities - was responsible for this observation. The lag time between start of stimulation and the start of milk ejection varies concerning to the actual degree of udder filling (Bruckmaier & Hilger, 2002), on average the milk ejection starting about 40 to 80 s after start of pre-stimulation. The

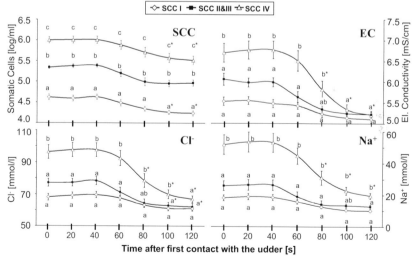

Figure 1. Patterns of SCC, EC, Na^+ and Cl in the SCC-Groups in relation to the milk fractions. Means ± SEM; n=20 cows; three milking times each cow; a, b, c different letters indicate significant differences between groups ($P < 0.05$); * indicate significant differences as compared to t=0s ($P<0.05$).

dilution of the cisternal milk fraction, an amount of about 20% of the totally stored milk (Pfeilsticker et al. 1996), was obviously the reason for the observed phenomenon.

In experiment 2 467 samples were analysed and classified as presented in table 1. EC, Cl and Na means between *SCC I* and *SCC IV* groups differed significantly in the first two sampled quarters, whereas means of EC, Cl and Na in *SCC I* and *SCC IV* were similar in quarter three and four.

Figure 2 presents exemplary the relationship between EC threshold level and the resulting sensitivity and specificity to distinguish between a SCC limit of 200.000 cells/ml.

In the first sampled quarter (RF), both sensitivity and specificity were rather high. With increasing sampling time the performance to detect elevated SCC decreased dramatically. A similar relationship was observed for Cl and Na (not shown).

Table 1. Analysis of SCC classes (n=6 cows; 20 consecutive milking times each cow).

quarter	sequence of sampling	number of observations					test on difference (SCC I vs. SCC IV; P = 0.05)		
		total	SCC I	SCC II	SCC III	SCC IV	EC	Cl⁻	Na⁺
RF	1	118	56	26	22	14	< 0.001	< 0.001	< 0.001
RR	2	114	56	17	15	26	< 0.001	< 0.001	< 0.001
LF	3	116	64	23	17	12	0.1779	0.3431	0.2422
LR	4	119	104	4	8	3	0.7673	0.1733	0.6255
total		467	280	70	62	55	< 0.001	< 0.001	< 0.001

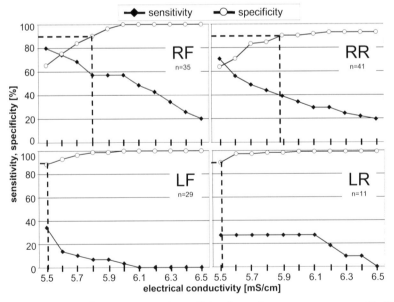

Figure 2. Quarter specific sensitivity and specificity dependent on a quarter specific EC threshold to detect a SCC limit of 200,000 cells/ml. Sampling sequence: right front (RF)=1, right rear (RR)=2, left front (LF)=3, left rear (LR)=4; dotted line represents a specificity level of 90%.

In table 2, quarter specific thresholds at a specificity of 90 % and their corresponding sensitivities are grouped for the three evaluated parameters and each quarter. In the best case (RF) it is possible to detect about 80 % of all quarter milk samples with more than 200,000 cells/ml using Na^+ measurement.

The sensitivities for the other quarters (between 42 % and 52 %) are not satisfactory. The EC values for all samples yielded a detection rate of 48 %, which is insufficient (also confirmed by Hamann & Zecconi (1998)). The inclusion of Cl and Na values improved the sensitivity to 64 % all over the quarters.

Table 2. Quarter specific thresholds and sensitivities for the EC, Cl, Na at a specificity of 90 % and a limit for SCC of 200,000 cells/ml (n=6 cows; 20 milkings per cow).

quarter	sequence of sampling	threshold (to get 90% specificity)			sensitivity (at 90% specificity)				number of observations with >200.000 cells/ml
		EC [mS/cm]	Cl- [mmol/l]	Na+ [mmol/l]	EC	Cl-	Na+	combination of EC, Cl-, Na+	
RF	1	5,8	64	21	57%	63%	80%	80%	35
RR	2	5,9	77	29	39%	24%	32%	42%	41
LF	3	5,5	56	15	35%	35%	31%	52%	29
LR	4	5,5	54	14	27%	46%	36%	46%	11
total		5,6	62	19	48%	52%	54%	64%	116

Conclusion

EC, Cl and Na can be a useful indicator for on-line detection of elevated SCC, when milk samples of cisternal milk before the start of alveolar milk ejection are available. Transferring the achieved results to automatic milking, the routine for taking samples used to determine the udder health needs special consideration with respect to sample time.

References

Bruckmaier, R. M. and Hilger, M. (2001). Milking ejection of dairy cows at different degrees of udder filling. -In: Journal of Dairy Research 68, pp 369-376

Burvenich, C. (1983). Mammary blood flow in lactating goats under several physiological and pathological (mastitis) conditions. Ph. D. thesis, University of Gent

deMol, R.M, Woldt, W.E. (2001) Application of fuzzy logic in automated cow status monitoring. In: Journal of Dairy Science 84, pp 400-411

Hamann, J. ; Zecconi, A. (1998). Evaluation of the electrical conductivity of milk as a mastitis indicator. -In: Bulletin of the International Dairy Federation 334, pp 5-22

Hillerton, J. E. (2000): Detecting mastitis cow-side. -In: Proceedings of the National Mastitis Council Annual Meeting, pp 48-53

Nguyen, D.D. and Neville, M.C. (1998). Tight junction regulation in the mammary gland. -In: Journal of Mammary Gland Biology and Neoplasia 3, pp 233-246

Olmos, P.R., Echevarria, J., Etxebarria, B., Castresana, J. M., Gallastegui, A. (1992). Determination of sodium in milk powders in baby feed using ion-selective electrodes -In: Alimentaria 230, pp 61-65

Ontsouka, C. E., Bruckmaier R. M., Blum J. W. Fractionized milk composition during removal of colostrums and mature milk In: Journal of Dairy Science. in press

Pfeilsticker, H. U.; Bruckmaier, R. M.; Blum, J. W. (1996). Cisternal milk in the dairy cow during lactation and after preceding teat stimulation. -In: Journal of Dairy Research 63, pp 509-515

Randell, A.W., Linklater, P.M (1972). The Rapid Analysis of Cheddar Cheese. 1. The Determination of Salt Content Using an Electrode Specific for Chloride Ion -In: Australian Journal of Dairy Technology 27, pp 51

Schulz, M. E.; Sydow, G. (1957). Die „chloridfreie" Leitfähigkeit von Milch und Milchprodukten (The chloride-free measurement of electrical conductivity of milk and milk products). -In: Milchwissenschaften 5 (12), pp 174-184

Smith, K. L. (1995). Standards for somatic cells in milk: physiological and regulatory. -In: IDF Mastitis Newsletter 144/21, pp 7-9

Wendl, G.: Schön, H.(2002). Techniques for cattle husbandry- In: Yearbook Agricultural Engineering (14), Ed.: J. Matthies et al., Münster: Landwirtschaftsverlag GmbH, pp 175 - 181

Acknowledgements

This project was funded by the Bavarian Ministry of Agriculture and Forestry (StMLF) and the Hanns Seidel Foundation e.V. Munich.

Authors index

Aerts, J.-M. 27
Altieri, G. 39
Antler, A. 113
Antman, A. 113
Artmann, R. 15
Bekkering, J. 23
Berckmans, D. 27
Berger, A. 131
Bollhalder, H. 87
Brandt, H. 23
Bruckmaier, R.M. 173
Chesmore, E.D. 33
Colangelo, A. 39
Di Renzo, G.C. 39
Donald, G. 93
Edan, Y. 67, 113
Edirisinghe, A. 93
Eichhorn, K. 131
Firk, R. 99
Frost, A.R. 47
Gebresenbet, G. 53
Geers, R. 53
Giuratrabocchetti, G. 39
Golden, B.L. 167
Gysi, M. 87
Haapala, H.E.S. 59
Halachmi, I. 67
Harms, J. 75
Hendriks, M.M.W.B. 149
Henry, D. 93
Hoy, T. 23
Ikeda, Y. 81
Ipema, A.H. 125
Jahns, G. 81
Junge, W. 99
Kaufmann, O. 161
Kaufmann, R. 87
Kelly, R. 93
Ketelaars, J.J.M.H. 149, 155
Kornet, J.G. 149
Krieter, J. 99
Lake, M. 33
Langbein, J. 105, 131
Livshin, N. 113
Lokhorst, C. 125, 149, 155
Maltz, E. 67, 113
Manteuffel, G. 105, 143
Matza, S. 113

Moallem, U. 67
Morio, Y. 81
Nishizu, T. 81
Nürnberg, G. 105
Oldham, C. 93
Ordolff, D. 119
Parsons, D.J. 47
Pompe, J.C.A.M. 125
Puppe, B. 143
Rademacher, I.F. 137
Robertson, A.P. 47
Sato, K. 81
Scheibe, K.M. 131
Schellberg, J. 137
Schofield, C.P. 47
Schön, P.C. 143
Schut, A.G.T. 149, 155
Shadduck, J.A. 167
Stacey, K.F. 47
Stamer, E. 99
Streich, W.J. 131
Talling, J.C. 33
Unrath, J. 161
Van Buggenhout, S. 27
Van de Water, G. 53
Van Driel, K.S. 33
Wantia, S.J.M. 125
Weiss, D. 173
Wendl, G. 75, 173
Whittier, J.C. 167
Wiedemann, M. 173
Yoon, C.S. 33

Keyword index